ON MY
WAY
BACK
TO
YOU

ON MY WAY BACK TO YOU

One Couple's Journey through
Catastrophic Illness to Healing and Hope

SARAH CART

WITH GLENN PLASKIN

Forefront
BOOKS

Published by Forefront Books, Nashville, Tennessee.
Distributed by Simon & Schuster.

Library of Congress Control Number: 2023919054

Print ISBN: 978-1-63763-251-2
E-book ISBN: 978-1-63763-252-9

Cover Design by George Stevens, G Sharp Design LLC
Interior Design by PerfecType, Nashville, TN
Printed in the United States of America

*To organ donors and their families for enabling miracles,
the medical personnel who find a path forward and pave it when
possible, and the angels among us who raise us up on the darkest days.*

Certain thoughts are prayers. There are moments when, whatever be the attitude of the body, the soul is on its knees.
—Victor Hugo, *Les Misérables*

Contents

Preface

L ife is hard, messy, beautiful, unpredictable . . . and fragile.

In our prime, it seems as if we are in the best of health with everything going our way. We feel invincible. Whole days, weeks, months, years race by, and in our haste, we don't fully appreciate our glowing health until something goes awry. As one season of life evolves into the next, a physical challenge suddenly arises to test us in every possible way.

That's what happened to my husband, Ben. And that's what this book is about: Ben's experience facing a life-threatening illness and coping with a medical crisis that appeared out of nowhere—one that almost killed him. Like collapsing dominoes, each setback toppled into the next, nearly crushing us both.

It's one thing to know objectively that there are no guarantees in this world; it's quite another to be challenged by that reality. We never know how long our loved ones will be with us. And there is certainly no promise that the health we enjoy this evening will be with us in the morning.

Although facing the fragility of life can be scary, it can also be empowering. It can help us remember to be grateful and cherish every day that comes our way.

As you'll read, my husband, Ben, just past his midfifties, was irrepressibly healthy and energetic until, suddenly, he wasn't. Throughout the more than three years during which his health declined precipitously, I kept a journal and took meticulous notes at every medical appointment.

Documenting the details of his condition—which was critical for communicating with his various doctors and specialists, as well as for understanding the way it affected us and our four sons—provided a means of grappling with the fear. Getting my thoughts and feelings on paper proved therapeutic. The catharsis of writing down what we were going through gave me the illusion that, if we could partially control it, perhaps we might tame the beast that was attempting to devour us. And there were many days when that illusion was the best thing—the only thing—we had going for us.

And as you'll see, during our odyssey of seemingly endless medical crises and appointments, I had to come to terms with the all-too-real possibility of Ben's imminent death. What kept me going? How did I handle the role of 24-7 caregiver for a husband who had previously been so independent and strong? When Ben's issues landed him in the ER less than two weeks after the world went into lockdown because of the newly declared COVID-19 pandemic, how did we unravel the tangle of unanticipated complications that followed?

Until we found ourselves in the thick of this battle, I'd always considered our life to be one of gloriously controlled chaos. We were blessed with four sons and four grandchildren, loving extended family and friends spread across the country and the world, frequent houseguests, lots of dogs, and an exceedingly comfortable life, thanks to Ben's thirty-year relationship with his terrific business partner, Mark Depew, and the small oil and gas company they built. But then our world turned upside down, and just as Ben's issues reached their most dire stage, the outside world turned upside down too.

I offer you this story not because you will necessarily be interested in our particular saga but because life *is* hard and messy and unpredictable, and chances are high that ultimately each of us will face challenges we never imagined—challenges that will knock us to our knees just when we least expect them. We never know how resilient we can be until we are tested. My wish is that, in such a moment, this book radiates hope and lights a way forward.

So in the pages ahead, you will discover some of the lessons I've learned about gratitude, patience, grace, and finding peace. About allowing yourself to be vulnerable. About finding strength in the realization that you are *not* alone. About fortifying your sense of independence while being, more than ever, open to and mindful of the abundance of support and love that surrounds you.

You'll also see how the miracles of modern science and communication can (and sometimes cannot) fully support a profoundly ill patient and the patient's loved ones.

Ben and I have been unbelievably blessed, thanks in no small part to a suffering family who, in what must have been their darkest hours, graciously and generously turned their loss into our miracle. Life *is* fragile and beautiful. These days, when people ask how Ben is doing, I am awed and grateful to be able to say, "He is doing so well that on occasion, he annoys me. And. It. Is. Wonderful."

Oliver Wendell Holmes Sr. wrote, "Death tugs at my ear and says, 'Live, I am coming.'" My hope is that Ben's story—our story—inspires you to live and treasure each moment.

Sarah Cart
Key Largo, Florida
April 2024

Prologue

BEFORE

That my husband, Ben, was dealing with something strange first became apparent in the fall of 2016, at the conclusion of a cousin's wedding on a beautiful afternoon in Ohio. Since forever, in any situation where other people might clap in appreciation, Ben would audibly demonstrate his enthusiasm by placing the tips of his pinkie and forefinger in the corners of his mouth, tucking them under the sides of his tongue. Then, with a quick exhale, he'd produce an earsplitting whistle. But this time, as the young bride and groom turned from the altar to be introduced to the congregation for the first time as husband and wife and everyone began to applaud, I realized that Ben was holding his right hand with his left even as he executed the expected blare.

"What's up with that?" I whispered. "A two-handed whistle?"

"Oh, that's to get my fingers close enough together; they've been swelling off and on lately."

Then, following the wedding weekend and with the arrival of cool weather, Ben also began showing a marked sensitivity to temperature changes. As he explored the woods around our cabin in Pennsylvania's Pocono Mountains, his fingers and toes would turn a sickly blue or even a deathly white. Occasionally he'd comment that his ankles were swollen. So when we got back to our primary residence, in Florida, and went for our flu shots in mid-November, I asked our longtime friend and general practitioner, Dr. Carlos Smith, if the swelling was cause for concern.

"Might be. Just in case, let's skip Ben's flu shot today and do some blood work instead."

Over the following weeks, Ben made numerous trips to Carlos's office and underwent a battery of tests. Finally, in December, Carlos called us both in to share the results. It appeared that Ben was facing a significant and progressive autoimmune condition, although Carlos wanted to leave the final identification up to a specialist.

He counseled us that Ben's constellation of symptoms would best be evaluated by a rheumatologist, so three months after that two-handed wedding whistle, we drove seventy-five minutes north to Cleveland Clinic Florida (hereafter referred to as "the clinic," or CCF) to meet with Dr. Hossam Elzawawy, who diagnosed Ben's predicament as systemic sclerosis.

Systemic sclerosis is an umbrella condition under which, Dr. Elzawawy explained, several other conditions are classified, from scleroderma (a hardening of the skin, sometimes damaging internal organs and joints in the process) to Raynaud's disease (the circulation problem affecting Ben's hands and feet) to dangerous edema (swelling) and much more.

"There is no cure," he stated. "The treatment is symptom by symptom." If it were to get to Ben's lungs, that would be bad.

As a concept, the disease was overwhelming, but we were eager for instructions on how best to stay ahead of it. Dr. Elzawawy told Ben that making sure his hands and feet stayed warm was important for keeping the Raynaud's at bay. ("Wear gloves. Wear socks. Don't let your extremities get cold or you'll risk amputation.") And he prescribed what seemed like massive quantities of immunosuppressants, remarking that the dosages would be changed as necessary, dictated by the results of blood work to be conducted every couple of months. Then, having taken our measure and advising us to stick to a healthy diet, he concluded that first consultation by cautioning us not to obsess about the test results that had put us on the path to Ben's diagnosis.

"Those numbers are what they are; you cannot change or improve them."

We were, however, to keep a diary of Ben's Raynaud's and swelling episodes. Tracking his diet might also be helpful. Follow-up appointments were scheduled for March and May of 2017, and we were advised to find a pulmonologist and get a baseline CT scan of Ben's lungs.

Ben Reflects

At first, I didn't believe anything could be seriously wrong. I thought a rheumatologist was for old people. A vivid memory from that first appointment with Dr. Elzawawy is the moment when he put some oil on the beds of my fingernails, then stuck them under a big microscope to see the little tiny capillaries up close. Some of them were not working, indicating defective circulation. That was the start of it all.

I'm pretty scientific rather than emotional. So at first I was somewhat detached about it. I'm not going to say I was in denial, but I wasn't seriously worried yet. Like, okay, I got this, so what do we do? It wasn't so dire. But then Dr. Elzawawy looked at me and said, "You're in the beginning of a five-year decline," and he put me on some immunosuppressants to slow the disease down.

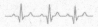

We were flummoxed as we tried to identify what, exactly, this systemic sclerosis was and how it would progress. How could Ben, who'd just turned fifty-eight, have some rare disease typically diagnosed in women between the ages of thirty and fifty? What was this bizarre syndrome that, according to the doctors and articles on the internet, causes the body to produce too much collagen?

Collagen? Really? Given the First World's ongoing obsession with youth, and living as we are in the midst of this "sixty is the new forty" era, was it even possible that there could *be* such a thing as too much collagen? Wasn't that touted as a crucial ingredient in supplements and lotions that counteract aging and are vital to the pursuit of wellness and beauty? What would collagen accumulating in various tissues, joints, and organs even mean?

Besides, what was the point of Ben taking so many pills when he wasn't in any real pain? He merely had to endure the occasional inconvenience of swollen fingers or tingling feet as they regained their color after going all white or blue—although even just a five-degree drop in temperature (experienced, say, when he entered an air-conditioned room) could trigger the color change.

Our incredulity was followed by what was perhaps our most naive question. At the March appointment, after telling Dr. Elzawawy that we customarily spend early June through late November at our cabin in the Poconos, he suggested that we proactively find a Pennsylvania rheumatologist and schedule a midsummer appointment.

"Is that really necessary?" we wondered aloud. We thought rheumatologists dealt with joints and skeletal issues. Weren't Ben's issues circulatory in nature?

"It may indeed be necessary," Dr. Elzawawy replied. "Make an appointment just in case. Because in the northeastern United States, rheumatologists can get very busy."

Seeing our raised eyebrows, he added, "You can always cancel if you find you don't need it. Ben's case is not medically complicated. Yet."

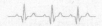

Credit to Dr. Elzawawy: we scheduled a July appointment with Dr. Julio Ramos, a Pennsylvania rheumatologist, and as it turned out, Ben did in fact need it. And many others throughout the seasons to follow.

CHAPTER 1

In the Beginning

July 2017—November 2018

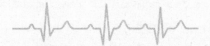

The changes brought about by Ben's systemic sclerosis were subtle at first. He didn't complain and frequently refrained from mentioning any new development until it was so far along that he knew it couldn't be his imagination. But as the months passed, he began to comment on various aches and pains, first in his joints, then in his tendons. From there, his autoimmune issues began to expand their horizons.

He suffered sudden and severe hearing loss, especially notable and frustrating since he was already hard of hearing. GERD (gastroesophageal reflux disease) and heartburn followed as the disease migrated from one bodily system to another. Between the Fourth of July and Labor Day of 2017, Ben dropped from 195 to 170 pounds as the muscles in his gastrointestinal tract came under fire, making absorbing nutrition a challenge. Through it all, in consultation with Drs. Elzawawy and Ramos, some medications were added, others were discontinued, and dosages were adjusted.

Yet despite an expanding list of limitations, Ben continued to pursue his passions, from treading softly along the edges of a trout stream stalking brookies, rainbows, and browns with a fly rod; hauling a small one-man canoe and binoculars to a remote pond for an afternoon's exploration; and traipsing through the woods to track the movements of birds, deer, or bear up North, to exploring the mangroves for snook and redfish and the flats for bonefish down South.

Ben Reflects

I never had a health problem—ever. I was always active, between my work and my outdoor activities, although I didn't much enjoy exercising for its own sake. Still, I wasn't afraid to get dirty or go out and do something physical that I felt like doing. And if it wore me out, that was great. My favorite form of exercise always involved being outdoors, which is why hunting and fishing and even just walking became so important. I also played ice hockey on a team called the Rustheads. And as a couple, Sarah and I were quite active. Anytime you saw us out together, we were likely to be dancing.

Ben has always loved the natural world. He grew up in rural New Jersey, across the road from his paternal grandparents' house, in the midst of beautiful gentlemen's farms with rolling hills and breathtaking views, and often wandered off to look for critters in the fields, the ponds, and the woods. He was reportedly obsessed with creepy-crawly stuff even before he learned to walk. Apparently, at the age of three, he once placed a colander over a copperhead. If it was cool and interesting, he wanted and needed to touch it—not to hurt it but to "check it out" and learn about it. The first books he remembers reading are field guides to reptiles—he memorized every snake listed.

Forever favorably compared to the Energizer Bunny and Tigger from *Winnie-the-Pooh*, to this point Ben had always been a man of seemingly boundless energy and limitless curiosity. He also appeared constitutionally suited to be a camp counselor: in Pennsylvania, whenever young children were around, he could be easily coaxed into providing lessons on how to catch and hold an eft, a toad, or a northern banded water snake. In Florida, he would lead hermit crab searches and night explorations in search of geckos and owls—or occasional midnight escapades to fly-fish for tarpon.

In fact, although my childhood activities when I was visiting my grandparents in Pennsylvania had always been related to swimming and canoeing, Ben's had forever run along the lines of fly-fishing, skeet shooting, and trapshooting. (His hearing issues have a lot to do with genetics, but they were exacerbated by an incident that took place on a shooting range when he was around twelve and wasn't wearing enough ear protection.) When he and I got engaged, his mother gave me a fly rod and reel with a note that advised, "Learn how to use these; I have found them to be helpful in ensuring a good marriage when marrying into the Cart family."

During that summer of 2017, Ben continued to spend eight to ten hours out of every twenty-four at his desk or on the phone with Mark, his business partner of thirty years. Ben and Mark's small Ohio company, Petrox, which they established at the end of 1986, had grown and thrived over the course of the ensuing decades.

The business focused on acquiring old oil and gas wells. Many of the individual wells had been running for years and were slowing down. But with some TLC, timing changes, chemical treatments, and other adjustments, many of them became efficiently productive again. As for those that were too old to resuscitate, Ben and Mark would work closely with the Ohio EPA to shut them in and pull the pipe, which opened additional marketing opportunities as they sold off the used equipment.

While there were some tough years at the beginning, over time the partners were nurtured by some generous benefactors, and hard work and determination helped them grow the company to the point where it sustained a comfortable midwestern lifestyle for both our family and Mark's, each of which was eventually blessed with four children.

Ben and Mark worked so closely together, talking every day, that they seemed like brothers—and still do, even though these days they only talk once every couple of months or so. I often remarked to people that they were "the happiest married couple I know"—their disagreements were few, and they negotiated remarkably well with, and on behalf of, each other. It didn't hurt that Mark naturally speaks loudly enough to be heard a mile away, a good fit with Ben's damaged hearing.

Eventually, Ben's role became more office-oriented while Mark's focused on the field. That meant Ben was able to work from almost anywhere, thanks to cell phones, laptops, and Wi-Fi—a flexibility that proved valuable because, once we became empty nesters, we also became snowbirds, finally able to follow the warm weather south in the winter and return north again in the summer. Those shifts accommodated both Ben's lifelong love of fishing and my visceral need to have a home near the water, a relic of my having grown up with a panoramic view of the Hudson River in Westchester County, New York.

Thus as the summer of 2017 progressed, Ben continued to work at his desk as he always had and we maintained our daily routines as well as we could. But increasingly, he would experience some new medical symptom that demanded attention. There were spontaneous nosebleeds; there was trouble swallowing and general ennui. At one point, simply opening his mouth wide enough to take a bite of a modest peanut-butter-and-jelly sandwich proved challenging. He developed carpal tunnel syndrome, and shooting pains in his tendons made it difficult to walk any appreciable distance. He tried physical therapy to stave off the encroaching limitations on his ability to get around. He had trouble grasping and casting a fishing rod and holding and firing a shotgun. He spent increasing amounts of time sleeping, and his blood pressure, already low, began to trend downward.

One incident that took place shortly before his autoimmune issues were conclusively identified illustrates how steep Ben's decline had become in barely more than six months.

It was early January in the Keys, and I was cleaning up after dinner. My cell phone rang—*probably a telemarketer* was my first thought. But the caller ID showed that it was a friend who lived nearby.

"Hey, Heather! What's up?"

"Is Ben there?" She sounded rushed and giddy.

"He's upstairs. Do you want to talk to him?" I headed into the hall. "No—there's not time. He needs to get over here. There's a snake!"

"Where?"

Even though we were a floor apart, and despite his impaired hearing, the urgent pitch of my voice got Ben's attention. He emerged from his office, and our eyes met.

"Snake," I mouthed, and he bounded down the stairs two by two. He slipped his feet into his Crocs, grabbed the keys to his Yamaha C3 scooter, and headed into the garage before he knew the details.

Heather continued, "We were on our way back from dinner. I'm driving, and Chuck says, 'Don't hit that log!' But it wasn't a log: it was a big fat snake crossing right in front of us!"

"We're on our way. Where should we meet you?"

"By the main entrance to the park—it slipped into the edge of the trees there. Hurry!"

Our friends and neighbors in the Poconos know not to share stories of timber rattlers that have suffered lead poisoning at the wrong end of a shotgun or rubber poisoning under the tire of an SUV, and Ben is always disappointed when he learns of a snake that wasn't left alone in its native environment. "They were here first," he likes to observe. "The rattlers are polite enough to warn us away; they deserve our respect." Our friends and neighbors in the Keys who've been made aware of his passion indulge him whenever the opportunity arises.

I hopped on the back of the scooter, and by the time we'd found Heather and Chuck, they'd been joined by Jim, one of our community's security guards, whose job description extends to ensuring that any invasive critters that show up in the neighborhood are properly dispatched. Heather and Chuck were using the flashlights on their phones. I added mine to the mix, and Jim swept the ground with an industrial-size light that had a broader beam.

Skipping the niceties, Ben demanded, "Where'd you last see it?"

"It went into the trees right here," Heather said, then Ben disappeared. The only trace of him was the sweep of his own high-end military-grade pocket flashlight, casting its beam over the ground, through the lower branches, and up the tree trunks into the overstory.

"Wait! What's he doing?" Heather sounded panicked.

"Jim, you need to get in there with him and make sure he's okay," Chuck said. Jim looked at me, hoping I'd say he didn't have to go.

"It's up to you," was all I could offer before Ben commanded, "Sarah, get into the park and watch the pathway. If the snake comes out, keep it from getting to the water or back to the trees."

Having first experienced this decades ago, when we were in college, I'd learned it's just easiest to play along. So I moved quickly, Heather and Chuck in my wake.

Then Ben's flashlight went dark.

Jim, in alarm, said, "Mr. Cart! What the—"

Then we heard a tussle and a scrabbling and a thump or two in the scrub that separated the park from the road.

Heather asked, "What's happening?" followed by Chuck's "Is he going to hurt himself?

Does he know what he's doing?"

I responded, "Don't worry; he's fine. This is good for him. He's going to catch it and bring it out for you to see."

As promised, right on cue, Ben emerged, beaming, with an eight-foot Burmese python draped across his shoulders. Standing there illuminated by our flashlights, the joy on his face rivaled that of a little boy on Christmas morning.

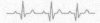

Because Ben insisted on looking at every part of his situation through rose-colored glasses, various projects that he and I would never have hesitated to tackle and solve together began to fall to me alone. I was devastated the first time I had to ask some friends for help—it was simply to rearrange a set of twin beds, but Ben wasn't physically up to the teamwork required. And as our roles shifted, I also became the one logging the majority of miles at the wheel, whether we were going to his doctor appointments or making our semiannual change of latitude.

He found that lying down became uncomfortable, not only because of heartburn but also because his skin was becoming so sensitive that he couldn't tolerate bedcoverings. When his college roommates—Dan the banker, Pete the veterinary pathologist, and Jon the cardiovascular surgeon—and their wives (Hitomi, Jillian, and Carrie) joined us for our traditional once-a-year Poconos house party weekend, the guys moved a recliner into his office so he could try sleeping relatively upright.

Meanwhile, the roster of medical professionals, both north and south, grew. GP: Check. Rheumatologist: Check. Pulmonologist: Check. Gastroenterologist: Check. Audiologist: Check. Physical therapist: Check. Nutritionist: Check. And despite his growing list of ailments and the expanding roster of professionals, Ben was fascinated by the science involved with each new development.

As we became more intimate with the disease that was turning Ben's world upside down, we repeatedly gave thanks that the insurance-defined diagnosis written in his chart, "Raynaud's disease without gangrene," included the word "without." We dreaded the possibility that one day that word might be deleted.

Then, in addition to all the tests and procedures, late in the spring of 2018, Dr. Elzawawy wrote a prescription for an ADA (American Disabilities Act) placard that would entitle Ben to use handicapped parking. My heart broke.

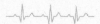

Ben and I were teenage sweethearts—we met when I was a freshman and he was a sophomore at Williams College, in Massachusetts. After he graduated, he secured a job with the oilfield services division of Dow Chemical, which began with an eighteen-month training program: six months working offshore in Louisiana, followed by six months working on shallow oil and gas wells around Youngstown, Ohio, and concluding with six months in an office in Tulsa, Oklahoma. In the midst of all that, I graduated, and just before his stint in Tulsa began, we got married. As we drove away from our reception, the wedding guests serenaded us with a rendition of "Oklahoma!"

With his training program behind him, Ben was assigned to return to Youngstown, and we settled in the nearby town of Poland, registered in 1796 as "Town 1, Range 1" of the Connecticut Western Reserve. In 1983, our first son, James, was born, and fourteen months later, in 1984, our second son, William, arrived. By the middle of 1985, we had bought a beautiful house with a fenced-in yard. The following year, Ben and Mark started Petrox, and Ben took over our basement for office space.

In 1989, we welcomed our third son, Ted; our youngest, Benjamin, was born in 1991.

Life was busy: I first worked part time writing for the local paper in Poland and doing PR for the Youngstown Playhouse, then I got a full-time job in the marketing department of a local architecture and engineering firm. When Ted was born, I went back to part-time work, writing for the Society section of Youngstown's daily paper, *The Vindicator*. Meanwhile, in addition to our jobs, Ben and I served on various boards—at church, at the Montessori school our boys attended, at the local hospital, the village council, and Junior League. We referred to our day-to-day lives as "controlled chaos."

For many years we rented a cabin in the Poconos at the end of the summer, and then in 2006 we bought one of our own and started staying more often. We enjoyed going there as much as possible from early spring through fall, but the northern winters were wearing on us. Then at one point, I needed to travel to the Hudson Valley to do a significant favor for a friend in need. As repayment, she offered Ben and me the use of a condo in Florida. Work and family commitments kept us from taking advantage of that invitation for a couple of years, but when we finally did, I realized I was *done* with subzero temperatures. We'd lived in Poland for more than three happy decades, but the moment Benjamin, our youngest son, followed the three older boys to attend school on the East Coast, we became bona fide empty nesters. In 2010, we sold our house in Ohio and became residents of the Sunshine State.

As the summer of 2018 began, Ben and I looked forward to a new grand-baby, due to arrive in Massachusetts in July. She would be our fourth, all fathered by our son James. We also had been invited to two weddings a week apart in August—one in Truckee, on the California side of Lake Tahoe, and the other just south of Cleveland, Ohio—and a fall weekend engagement party in DC for Ben's nephew. Ben was excited about all four occasions.

And although he was horribly fatigued and lacked energy, he was hugely relieved that the debilitating pain in his joints and tendons had gradually and noticeably diminished since the start of the year. We hopefully wondered if some of the stories we'd heard about systemic sclerosis were proving to be true. According to one of them, after three to five years, for some patients, the symptoms seem to resolve themselves—not that any injuries he had incurred would miraculously disappear, just that the disease would back off a bit. He wasn't at the three-year mark—not even close—but . . . were we turning a corner?

Ben was even feeling strong enough to walk away from his desk an hour or two before sunset most afternoons to get out into the woods and fields surrounding our cabin. He would stay out until dark and take note of how the weather and the direction of the wind affected the daily feeding habits of various deer, bear, wild turkey, pheasant, and grouse. He spent eleven months a year, from afar and on-site, preparing and looking forward to doing his part to help cull those populations come fall, and I had a raft of recipes for venison and wild game.

Then he started to gain weight. We rejoiced. Perhaps his GI tract was coming back online!

At the end of July, we made a one-day there-and-back road trip to Massachusetts to see our newest granddaughter within hours of her birth, and then at the beginning of August, we flew to Nevada.

Tahoe was beautiful, but the start of our trip had been complicated by airline delays. Despite our best-laid plans, conceived to minimize travel time and allow Ben to adjust to the three-hour time difference (which affected his medication schedule), and being six thousand feet above sea level, we ended up flying a day later than originally scheduled, leaving home at 4:00 a.m. in the pouring rain. We struggled through several airports to make numerous connections and arrived with barely enough time to straighten our clothes before sitting down at a rehearsal dinner for the wedding party and dozens of out-of-town guests. Plus, the southwestern skies were hazy and heavily tinged with smoke as a result of an already active fire season in California. So from the moment we arrived, Ben was exhausted and instantly found himself in taxing circumstances, struggling to breathe. In addition, his ankles were badly swollen after all that sitting on planes and in airports.

In fairness to Tahoe, in the ten days leading up to our travels, Ben had begun to experience breathlessness even when simply walking up the steps to get into our house from his car, but neither he nor I had attributed that to anything but a string of lousy nights' sleep. Plus, as soon as he'd climb into our bed, he'd begin windmilling through the hours so that by morning his head would be where his feet should be, and every pillow had become his and his alone. Often the issue was so pronounced that either he would retire to the recliner in his office, or I would move to the guest room. When traveling circumstances provided us a bed to share, I'd end up getting a better night's sleep on the floor.

Fortunately, our lovely Tahoe wedding weekend accommodations included a pair of queen-size beds, and Ben was able to sleep late, rest comfortably, and nap through the afternoons. Still, except for a couple of hours at the rehearsal dinner and the gorgeous mountaintop wedding itself, for much of the weekend I was a solo act.

A Son Reflects: Benjamin

When I learned that my dad was unwell, my first reaction was general confusion. The prognosis or general outlook for systemic sclerosis didn't seem conducive to making predictions. In short, all the research I could find seemed to lead to the same conclusion: "It can be bad, or it can be not that bad—it really depends how things go." Given that, my initial response, before things took a turn for the worst, could best be described as a general sort of anxiety. It wasn't clear what systemic sclerosis would mean for him, but it was obviously a stressful thing.

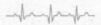

A week later, Ben slept as I drove us the six hours from northeastern Pennsylvania to Ohio for the wedding festivities of Mark's older son, Nathaniel. Again, we had budgeted extra travel time to allow Ben space to settle in and adjust before having to be social, and although we were a little surprised and unnerved at how little energy he had, we figured he was still catching up from the exhausting cross-country trip several days earlier. Again, his ankles, and now his calves, were badly swollen, even though we hadn't flown. We told ourselves it was the result of sitting in the car for so long.

Ben and Mark hadn't seen each other in person for ages, and I know Mark was stunned. Ben, ashen and a slow-moving shell of his former self, wouldn't commit to entering a cocktail party, brunch, luncheon, or dinner unless he could see exactly where he was going to be able to sit, and then he would go plant himself in that spot. I would make sure his drink glass stayed full and go through the buffet line for him. Yet Ben very much wanted to be there. The two entrepreneurs had been together through thick and thin for decades. We'd attended Mark and Brenda's wedding and had the joy of partying with the entire family, a fun crowd who enjoyed good music, and they remembered well that Ben and I love to dance.

Mark and Brenda were incredibly gracious hosts, treating us as dear relations and seating us among all their siblings throughout the weekend. My partner at the rehearsal dinner was Mark's brother-in-law Vivek, a critical-care physician who'd come in from Illinois. We had a lovely time catching up, and he was appropriately curious about Ben's condition. Then at the wedding reception, at the first hint of a favorite song, I stood up.

"Come on, Ben! You're feeling well enough for this, aren't you? Please?" He laughed as I dragged him into the reveling crowd.

Vivek watched us dancing. And witnessed Ben bow out before the end of the first chorus to take a seat.

Not wanting to pry, Vivek was sympathetic as he asked about Ben's shortness of breath. He carefully posed lots of other questions too. It was obvious: as a professional, he was seeing the worrisome details we were working hard to ignore. He suggested that Ben see a cardiologist as soon as I'd driven us back across Pennsylvania. He also gave us his business card and a list of tests to ask about. "Please know that I am happy to talk with you. Anytime. Do not hesitate to call me."

Benjamin Reflects

My dad was always an energetic guy. When we were growing up, he was always up early, sipping coffee and working at his desk in his basement home office. As a kid, I distinctly remember him being great at throwing a Frisbee and playing hockey at our local rink. Much more often, though, my dad's activity took the shape of hunting and fishing. It was sometimes frustrating for me and my brothers because our patience for those activities would wear out long before his did. When we were done for the day, he would have happily stayed out for hours longer.

And even in social situations, my father was always the type of guy to close out whatever function he was attending—dancing late into the night, sticking around till the end, chatting with friends—rather than ever pulling an Irish exit.

A Son Reflects: William

My dad has always been a very high-energy person. Maybe this was because of the three-plus pots of coffee he used to drink during the workday. I always described him as someone who lived on the balls of his feet. If he was talking to someone, that's where he'd put his weight; he'd lean slightly forward, excitedly telling a story or listening intently. We often had to wait in the car at church while he finished talking to people.

He played hockey, took care of the yard, and worked in the basement until all hours. He was up early and reading the Wall Street Journal when it was still dark. He was a bundle of energy for my entire childhood.

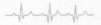

I drove us back to the Poconos on Sunday, and we got Ben to our GP in Scranton on Tuesday, having called Vivek on Monday to go over the questions we should ask. We also sought advice from Ben's college roommate Jon, the cardiovascular surgeon, who lived in Hartford, Connecticut.

We braced ourselves, but we still weren't prepared when Dr. Daniel Kasmierski pronounced the diagnosis: "Congestive heart failure."

Ben teared up; those had been the exact words on his grandfather's death certificate.

That was the reason Ben had gained so much weight so quickly. That was why he was so exhausted. That was why he was having trouble breathing.

That was why there was more swelling in his ankles than we'd ever seen before—and sometimes swelling in his calves and occasionally even above his knees.

We returned to our cabin in the woods, an hour away from the closest hospital, with a prescription for massive doses of diuretics. Ben dropped fifteen pounds in a week, at which point he was introduced to a cardiologist and an electrophysiologist.

Within moments of looking at Ben's echocardiogram, the cardiologist, Dr. Thomas Dzwoncyzk, declared, "This is not normal." He waited as I opened the spiral notebook where I'd been recording the details of Ben's medical adventures over the previous eighteen months, then he said, "Let me unpack it for you."

He proceeded in a clear, direct, and organized way to explain what was going on. The good news was that Ben had no weak valves and some "insignificant" leakage. The bad news was that his heart's electrical system was completely out of whack, meaning he had significant rhythm problems.

It was an immediate issue that could be addressed locally but, more important, needed to be addressed quickly. Beyond that, we needed to establish a relationship with a larger medical center that could better assess and meet Ben's evolving cardiac needs.

Because a few other tests were necessary and insurance needed to preapprove any treatment, Ben was sent home for the weekend with the simplest instructions we'd ever received:

"If *anything* goes wrong, get to the emergency room ASAP." I slept with one eye open for the next three nights.

Ben Reflects

There came a point when I couldn't finish a dance at a wedding. And a family member of the wedding party, who happened to be a doctor, looked at me and said, "You have a real heart problem; I can tell just by looking at you." That was a real wake-up call.

We had an awful moment two weeks after that when we met with a cardiologist. After running some tests, he came back in the room, and his face was gray as he told us both to sit down. He said, "I don't even know where to start." Then he explained the three ways my heart needed to get electrical impulses. Two of them were utterly broken, and the third one was about to break because of the tiny capillaries that weren't doing their jobs. He said, "You're going to need a pacemaker or you're going to die." And then he said, "So have a nice weekend, and we'll try to schedule the procedure for Tuesday and Wednesday of next week."

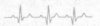

Barely a month after Vivek watched our retreat from the dance floor, Ben had a defibrillating pacemaker implanted.

We had badly miscalculated what Ben's systemic sclerosis was up to.

If, in fact, this even had anything to do with his systemic sclerosis. The doctors couldn't be sure. It was possible this was completely unrelated.

Meanwhile, we were instructed, were the pacemaker to give Ben what I dubbed "a correction" (or, in the technician's parlance, "a treatment"), we needed to call the doctor's office. If he got a second one, we were to call 911. That got our attention.

Ben and Mark agreed to begin negotiating his exit from the company the two of them had built. They had wisely spent a lot of effort and energy years earlier drawing up plans for and investing in disability insurance. The time to file a claim had come. Preliminary phone calls and emails were exchanged with the insurance company; it was going to be a complicated multistep process.

We also canceled plans to go to Washington, DC, for Ben's nephew's engagement party.

I found myself praying I'd be able to get Ben there twelve months later for the young man's wedding.

Fortunately, however, the immediate implementation of a nearly sodium-free diet, coupled with the pacemaker and various medications, enabled us to adopt a relatively stable new routine that also honored Ben's developing need to nap a lot.

With the pacemaker restoring a normal heart rhythm, Ben even felt strong enough to get back into the Pennsylvania wilderness, stepping into ground blinds or climbing up into tree stands—too often napping, but ultimately hunting the local wildlife and stocking our freezer with healthy lean free-range protein. The doctors were supportive of this obsession, but it made me anxious. I insisted that Ben text me as soon as he settled into each afternoon's position and again before he climbed out of the tree or stepped out of the blind to head to his truck and drive home. I made him "share location" on his phone and checked mine continually . . . just in case.

And I repeatedly hounded him about whether he was dressing warmly enough to keep the Raynaud's at bay. Despite that, over the course of a few weeks, another potentially serious problem appeared in the form of small ulcers on the tips of his fingers. These could be caused by the simplest things: the prick of a staple, a splinter of firewood, or even the stem of a grape.

He also developed ulcers on his toes and ankles. I suggested that perhaps the ones on his ankles were caused by a combination of cold weather and tight boots on his swollen feet. That was a possibility he did not want to entertain or discuss, because if we were to talk it through completely, I might insist that he stay in by the fireside every evening until the time came to head south again.

The more pressing problem, however, was that none of the wounds was healing.

CHAPTER 2

Curiouser and Curiouser

November 2018—March 2020

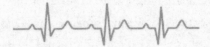

The self-contained Florida community where we live is tucked away in the northernmost section of the Keys; the salt air, the palms, the water views, and the flowers make it feel like the Caribbean. The preferred means of transportation around the community is a golf cart, even for those of us who don't golf, but there are also scooters and bicycles and plenty of cars and trucks, plus wonderful paths for walking. Because the two roads that lead to it are so far from any other towns (nineteen miles from the north, eleven miles from the south), there are security gates, a small medical center, a veterinarian, a gym, a couple of marinas, and a public safety and fire department. The people who have chosen to live and work this far from civilization have made a commitment to the community, and we are blessed to have them in our lives. We feel very lucky.

This was especially true immediately after Thanksgiving in 2018, when we returned to the Keys needing to add a southern cardiologist and electrophysiologist to Ben's matched north-and-south sets of doctors.

Fortunately, a cardiologist with Cleveland Clinic Florida, Dr. Howard Bush, visited patients at our community medical center often, so taking the first step in that direction proved relatively easy.

The next steps took longer.

Like the cardiologist and electrophysiologist in Scranton, Dr. Bush was baffled by Ben's case. Had the heart issues developed independently of the autoimmune disease? Or because of it?

While that felt like a chicken-and-egg question to us, the answer, if it could be found, would be helpful in determining the most appropriate treatment.

One option that had been under discussion since the summer's diagnosis of congestive heart failure was to do a cardiac biopsy, but none of the doctors expected that would provide any definitive answers. To move things forward as the year wound down, Dr. Bush explained that he would play the role of general contractor and arrange for Ben to meet with a succession of cardiology specialists through the first half of 2019 so they could work on solving the riddle.

That meant driving seventy miles to the Cleveland Clinic's campus in Weston, Florida, every six weeks or so, but we knew the drive; we'd simply combine some of the appointments with Ben's regular follow-ups with Dr. Elzawawy.

Then late one day shortly before Christmas, Ben determined that he was going to take advantage of one of the lovely benefits of living in Florida after decades of Midwest winters: the opportunity to go for a swim on a December afternoon and stretch in the warm water, easing his sore joints.

"I'm headed for the pool. Wanna join me?"

I was preparing some casseroles for holiday guests, and the kitchen looked like a war zone.

"Thank you, but if I stop now, it'll be hard to get back into this."

"Fine—I'll be back soon."

I resumed my chopping.

"Oh! Uh-oh. Um, I think maybe I'll go to the medical center instead."

Just as he was opening the door, one of his ankle ulcers ruptured. Wisely, he suggested that he take the golf cart to get some professional attention while I continue with those casseroles.

As it turned out, that ankle was so badly infected that it required an extended course of antibiotics; Ben wasn't going to be swimming for a while. He had been determined that I not get involved with bandages or any of the rest of it, and I was determined not to say, well, you know . . . that thing people say when they told you so.

Also, as 2018 drew to a close, Ben's sleep issues had come to include something like severe restless legs syndrome. He'd try to settle in for the night, and at the precise instant when he'd finally drop off, his muscles would spasm, and he'd wake himself up. So he'd go round and round in an endless loop of almost asleep–not asleep–almost asleep–not asleep. Consequently, staying awake and alert during daylight hours, whether he was working at his desk, watching a movie, sitting in the car, or conducting countless other activities of daily living, was proving to be a challenge. I'd return from errands to find him asleep at his desk or curled up on our bed napping, unable to concentrate on any task that took longer than a few minutes.

Ben Reflects

When I got the pacemaker, my life changed. I felt great again—so much better. But eventually, even the pacemaker couldn't help, because the muscles of my heart were failing. In other words, the pacemaker couldn't stop the hardening of my heart. It told the heart what to do, but the heart was getting less muscular every week.

On the cardiac front, the new year started with pulmonary function tests, an MRI, CT scans, echocardiograms, and increasingly interesting blood work.

The MRI was expected to be the most revealing, but between Ben's pacemaker, which required a technician from the manufacturer to be present in order to adjust it in real time, and his lousy circulation, which made it practically impossible for the technician to track Ben's pulse—a measurement that was crucial to performing the adjustment and enabling the imaging test to proceed—the first go-round had to be aborted, and rescheduling took months.

Plus, because of all the changes to his pharmaceutical cocktail as the systemic sclerosis progressed, and with his heart now needing medications of its own, Ben's blood pressure, which had always been low, devolved to a "normal" of about 85/55. We came to appreciate, but couldn't quite master, the fine art of keeping excess water off his frame so his heart wouldn't be taxed while still keeping his blood pressure high enough to prevent dizziness and fainting. Even with his pacemaker and diuretics, his legs and hands were swelling significantly.

His disability case file had finally been officially opened around Thanksgiving, but filling out the paperwork—a collection of authorization forms, statements from doctors, questionnaires, and cataloged lists of appointments, diagnoses, medications, and hospitalizations, among other things—was proving to be a major project beyond Ben's severely diminished capabilities.

Perpetually exhausted, he was unable to concentrate for more than ten minutes at a time.

Finally, he let me take on the major first step of the project, which consumed the last ten days of February. I'd needle him to stay awake long enough to dictate answers about the full scope of his duties and why he was no longer able to work. He'd then edit whatever I typed, finding it to be much simpler than staring at a blank sheet of paper and trying to figure out where to begin. I'd retype, and we'd redraft, until he was satisfied that the details were complete and accurate. I also transcribed his history of appointments and diagnoses from my spiral notebook, then produced several copies of the submission: one for Carlos and another for Dr. Elzawawy, along with the paperwork each of them needed to complete; one for the disability claims agent; one for our insurance representative; one for Mark; and one for our files. Shipping all those off was a tremendous relief.

After two months of procedures, Ben met with an electrophysiologist in March, a congenital cardiac disorders specialist in April, and in May, a heart-failure cardiologist. That spiral notebook was nearly full.

Luckily for us, college roommate Jon was just a phone call away to confirm and explain what we were learning. The consensus was that Ben's problems appeared to be primarily on the right side of his heart. Which, we were told, was good news (kinda), because that meant the issues weren't pulmonary or related to his lungs.

The bad news, however, was that it was rare and uncommon for the heart to deteriorate as rapidly and drastically as Ben's had.

Back to the good news: every doctor who met Ben found his case, with its unusual combination of heart failure, low blood pressure, and systemic sclerosis, intriguing.

Finally, the Cleveland Clinic team decided that a cardiac biopsy might not be able to tell them everything, but it would tell them something. The plan was to head north for the summer and fly back to the clinic for the procedure in July, making a one-night round trip to Fort Lauderdale with a stay at a hotel in Weston and not even going to our house in the Keys.

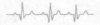

With our return to the Poconos in June of 2019, our lives took on the metaphoric aspect of climbing the endless staircase in that M. C. Escher lithograph *Relativity*. Although Ben was constantly, painfully exhausted, whenever he entered a doctor's office, he was upbeat and wide awake, asking questions, pushing for answers.

Jon proposed we consider going to his home turf, Hartford Hospital, a northern medical center with a major heart program. Basically, he wanted us to meet his associate (another heart-failure cardiologist) and let him work Ben up so he'd be an established patient . . . just in case. Although it was three hours away from our cabin, Hartford was an easy drive: a straight shot on the interstate, then three minutes on local streets. The other option was Philadelphia, which, while only two and a half hours away, involved several much busier highways and ended with stressful downtown traffic and a challenging parking garage.

While mulling Jon's suggestion, we also followed through and made appointments with all of Ben's Scranton physicians to bring them up to date. In late July, Dr. Dzwoncyzk, the cardiologist who'd "unpacked" the situation when Ben needed the pacemaker ten months earlier, reviewed what had been going on, including the results of the cardiac biopsy in Florida. Once more, his explanation was concise and clear: Ben's case was complicated.

He started by showing me that Ben's edema was even visible in his neck veins, a pulsing indicator of his failing heart. Then he counted additional causes for concern on his fingers, one by one.

- The left side of Ben's heart was moderately weak; the right side was enlarged.
- Ben had a leaky tricuspid valve, but because the enlarged right side was "like a balloon that's been inflated for quite a while and has lost its elasticity," a valve replacement wasn't a viable option; it would be putting good plumbing between bad joints.
- Most of the pharmaceuticals that would typically be used to stem heart failure wouldn't work for Ben because his blood pressure was already dangerously low (80/60 that day).
- And although there was a drug he could take, the results of which were often miraculous, that drug had dangerous side effects that increased mortality rates and therefore was considered an "end-stage" medication that could only be used for a couple of years. (I wanted Dr. Dzwoncyzk to stop "unpacking."

Immediately.) But, then he mentioned that this drug was considered "a bridge to transplant."

Wait. What?

Transplant?

We'd been avoiding that word, but now it was out there. And it
was unsettling. But more unsettling was the final thing Dr. Dzwoncyzk
unpacked: a note from Ben's Cleveland Clinic chart stating, "Patient's
systemic sclerosis may negate transplant candidacy."

Since Ben's initial autoimmune diagnosis, Jon had graciously agreed as
a good and dear friend to serve as sounding board and guide, helping
us understand all the various issues involved. He was flattered and more
than happy to do so, but he also warned us early on, "I consider you
family. I will *not* be your doctor."

Although theoretically we understood and fully supported what he
was saying, we now found ourselves, two and a half years in, standing
at the center of Jon's wheelhouse: as a cardiovascular surgeon, he had
performed hundreds of heart transplants.

It was time for a trip to Hartford to meet Jon's associate. Jon had told
Jason Gluck many stories about Ben, having known him for forty
years—not only his camp-counselor personality, his Tigger-like energy,
and his indefatigable Energizer Bunny determination when he has a goal
in mind but also his sheer grit in choosing to ignore the possibility of
negative outcomes and even his outrageous luck in backgammon (rolling
double sixes several times at the most critical junctures).

Before the appointment, Jason had thoroughly reviewed Ben's medical files and studied the results of all the procedures that had taken place
over the previous many months. After we spoke for a bit, he mentioned

his surprise at how strong Ben appeared in person—it belied everything in his chart. "That's a good thing," he added.

Plus, in his opinion and experience, "systemic sclerosis needn't be a barrier to transplant." In fact, Ben's treatment ought to be aggressive, especially since his systemic sclerosis was not likely to get any easier to manage.

"And you're not even sixty yet; you're young. You'll do better to get a transplant while you have good manual dexterity, because self-care will be important to your recovery, and manual dexterity might deteriorate if your autoimmune disease progresses further. Besides, I can see you've got the attitude necessary for the fight."

Jason noted that Ben had been retaining an increasing amount of water recently, albeit less than he had been accumulating before the pacemaker was implanted, and that since the Florida overnight trip, he'd experienced an even more drastic loss of energy. As an immediate remedy, Jason proposed a few days of IV therapy to get the water weight off Ben so at the very least, he could feel better.

Jason let us go back to the Poconos that afternoon so Ben could organize a few things on his desk, make some phone calls, and grab his iPad and chargers. But that same night, revitalized by the prospect of proactively responding to the matters at hand and with a good bit of adrenaline working in his favor, Ben drove (for the first time in months) back to Hartford to sleep (or at least stay in the guest room) at Jon and Carrie's house.

Late the next morning, he admitted himself to the hospital. He stayed for ten days and got a dramatic lesson in what it feels like to be at "dry weight" when the nurses siphoned twenty-five pounds of water from his system. He also got treated like a VIP because no one could figure out how, exactly, he was related to Jon. When the two were younger, they looked so much alike that people sometimes wondered if they were brothers, and the hospital staff was hyperaware of Jon's frequent visits.

Then too, none of them had ever witnessed Jon fetching ice for a patient before.

Because of the distance, I only visited every other day, but in addition to Jon and Carrie, our son William visited from New York, our son James drove southeast from northwestern Massachusetts, and Ben's sister came in from Boston to fill in on the days I missed. For the moment, Ben was safe and in a good place, surrounded by professionals much better able than I to address his issues.

William Reflects

When I learned about my father's illness, I was angry, scared, and confused. I was angry at him for smoking so many cigars. I was also angry and worried that his condition might have been caused by being around all those chemicals at work. I wanted a reason; I wanted to understand why this was happening.

I reacted by spending an immense amount of time with him, and those are some of my most precious memories. I came to the Poconos whenever I could and hunted with him in those years more than I did in any others. It was beautiful and meaningful to be with him in those moments as we bonded over our shared love for that place. It was also difficult.

I was deeply sad at times when I needed to drag an animal because I knew he simply could not do it. I remember a sporting clays competition in which he stopped shooting halfway through because his hands hurt too much, but he stayed to watch me finish. It was a wild experience to confront my father's mortality, particularly during those Poconos activities that are so deeply ingrained in all of us.

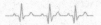

Naively, when Ben left for Hartford, I thought perhaps that before his return, he would be added to "the list" and the wait for a new heart would begin immediately.

I, and Ben, had a lot to learn.

The reality is that getting on any transplant center's list is a long and complicated process, consisting of visits to specialists and dozens and dozens of tests, evaluations, procedures, and follow-up appointments over the course of many months to assess every single aspect of a potential candidate's physical systems from top to bottom and inside out.

But when Ben was discharged from the hospital in Hartford, Jason and Jon made it clear that, in their educated opinion, a transplant was the only way we would have a future. They advised us to consider getting Ben on several transplant lists.

And we should start the process soon.

They were also brutally frank: unless we were planning to stay north through the coming winter, there wasn't enough time to complete the work necessary to get on their list before November. We'd end up having to commute north into the New England winter, which at the very least would stress Ben's Raynaud's. For the time being, we were going to have to agitate to get on the Cleveland Clinic's list in Florida, despite the systemic sclerosis, and immediately upon our return north in the spring, start running the hurdles in Hartford.

I hesitated. Was it ethical to push to be on more than one list?

Jon assured me, "Transplant teams are governed by strict protocols, and candidates are ranked according to need. If one heart could go to either of two patients, all things being equal, the one who's been listed longer gets first dibs, so the sooner Ben gets listed, the better. If and when he gets a heart, he comes off all the other lists, and everyone else moves up."

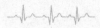

Throughout the fall, when friends asked, "How's Ben doing?" my answer was a variation on "When things are good, we can take them a day at a time. If they're really good, we can take them a whole week at a time. Sometimes we just take things hour by hour."

Thankfully, while I hadn't been able to get Ben to DC for that engagement party the previous year, we were able to get there for the October wedding. Everything to do with feting the honored couple, including the weather, was fairy-tale fabulous, spectacular, and wonderful. We got to spend time with extended family and almost all our immediate family; everyone except our youngest grandchild was there. Ben was awake and alert when he needed to be, including when he made a heartwarming toast at the rehearsal dinner.

But it was a bittersweet weekend, because for much of the time, I was once again part of a pair at a wedding but left on my own, whether it was to walk the Mall with the kids, visit with friends, or grab a bite to eat.

By the end of 2019, Ben's energy reserves were in negative territory, and a good night's sleep was a long-lost concept.

When we brought Dr. Bush up to speed on the August hospitalization, however, we were relieved and grateful that he agreed to shepherd Ben's efforts to get on the Cleveland Clinic's transplant list. The note in Ben's chart about systemic sclerosis negating transplant candidacy turned out to have been entered by a resident and was more of a question than a statement.

Simultaneously, though, while I felt the need to be loyal, I admitted to our four sons that in many ways dealing with their dad, a brilliant man who had started a wonderful company with an amazing partner more than thirty years earlier and sustained it through the decades, had become like trying to manage and live with a ten-year-old boy—a sweet, well-intentioned, adorable ten-year-old, but a ten-year-old nonetheless—with little capacity for long-range planning, remembering details, or considering consequences.

And the ulcers on his ankles were back. But, Ben assured me, they were under control, and he did not need my help.

From the get-go, 2020 was consumed with numerous medical appointments each week as we not only tried to keep Ben from losing any more ground but also continued to jump through whatever hoops Cleveland Clinic Florida had set up to ensure that all the doctors would eventually meet, confer, and agree that he was a viable transplant candidate.

In January alone, Ben had thirty-two appointments, a frequency that would continue as winter progressed. We hired a driver to spell me on occasion so I didn't have to go to all of them, but I went to most. Luckily, many were local, and for the ones that weren't, the clinic schedulers worked with us so that when we made the trek, our obligations would follow in succession, which made for long but productive days. Although many appointments were for physical therapy, and a few were with Carlos, the other two dozen or so included the dentist, audiologist, pulmonologist, sleep-disorder specialist, rheumatologist, and several cardiologists. There were also procedures and interviews involving Ben's sleep, kidneys, vascular function, and bone density along with X-rays, a carotid ultrasound, a visit to a wound clinic, and transplant education. Sometime soon, the clinic transplant team was going to require a colonoscopy as well, but the scheduling for that was proving problematic.

A Son Reflects: James

Dad's always been upbeat and active, from hosting neighborhood soccer games in our backyard to captaining (and sponsoring) hockey teams in our area. In fact, a few months before he went into the hospital, we all (me; my wife, Ashley; our four kids; and Mom and Dad) traveled together to Disney World. He was as upbeat as ever, but the physical shift was impossible to ignore. He was in a motorized wheelchair, following us around in the park, riding roller coasters he maybe shouldn't have been riding. I just remember seeing the dad I knew—strong, confident, funny, optimistic—looking feeble and tired. I didn't realize then, in February of 2020, that he was in as bad shape as he was, but I probably should have.

The circuslike pace kept up into March, even as there were alarming rumblings about a dangerous and highly contagious new virus making its way around the globe. People wondered whether it would reach the United States, and it was suggested that perhaps rather than shaking hands, we should greet one another by bumping elbows and refrain from greeting friends and family with hugs and pecks on the cheek.

I began to fantasize about having just twenty-four hours off. To sit quietly. To sleep soundly. To shower without being interrupted by a phone call regarding a test result or a pending appointment. To have a conversation with Ben that began with my saying something other than "What hurts? How can I help?"

But there's a reason they say, "Be careful what you wish for. You just might get it."

First thing on a Monday morning, I herniated a disk in my back. Not while working out or lifting anything heavy or doing anything outrageous . . . just while simply getting dressed.

Then I stupidly spent the day trying to power through the pain. When I finally called Carlos, late in the afternoon, he didn't mess around: I was transported by ambulance to a hospital in Miami for what turned into a four-night stay.

Several times a day, I would be wheeled on a gurney to another test in the far reaches of the facility, then back to my room. I was too high on pain medication to do anything more than stare at the television, receiving a primer on what little was known of the mystery virus creeping through the country. Friends kept an eye on Ben, who, because of his autoimmune status, couldn't visit. Although we could FaceTime once or twice a day, that wore me out quickly.

Then, late on the afternoon of day four, with all the test results in, the doctors proposed an epidural. It was miraculous: the pain evaporated within hours. I took a shower on my own that night, and the next day I called an Uber for a ride home, a bit worn out but hugely relieved to have avoided surgery.

My discharge instructions: No heavy lifting. No driving for a few weeks.

So now Ben made all his trips to the Cleveland Clinic by car service. In early March, although he had several evaluations still outstanding and was not yet eligible to be on the transplant list, we met with Debbie, the nurse assigned as Ben's transplant coordinator. In a bit of foreshadowing, she apologized for wearing a mask throughout the appointment and commented that she knew it looked strange, but she had a scratchy throat and didn't want to risk transmitting any germs; one thing working with the transplant team and patients had taught her was the importance of proceeding with an abundance of caution.

Benjamin Reflects

In 2020, when I finally grasped my father's worsening health issues and his need for a heart transplant, I remember how thoroughly this terrible news blended into the overall horrors of the world at that time. It was the peak of pandemic confusion, and we were already scared. Now suddenly there was an even bigger reason to be stressed out. I was really worried that COVID would be a major player in his health issues. I was waiting to get a call from my mom along the lines of "You need to get down here." Like everyone at the time, I generally felt helpless—but with a generous serving of even more helplessness on top of what was already there.

That afternoon, each of us signed clinic paperwork indicating that we understood that were Ben to become a transplant candidate and, we hoped, an eventual recipient, we would be taking on huge responsibilities, from compliance with all medical treatments to financial obligations to my role as his social support now and forever, doing whatever was necessary to build and maintain his health.

As we departed, Debbie presented us with a loose-leaf book entitled *Your Guide to Health and Recovery: Heart Transplant*. I flipped quickly through the tabbed sections: "Introduction to Heart Transplant," "Your Hospital Stay," "Your Recovery," "Medications," and "Living a Healthy Lifestyle." Debbie recommended we make time to work through it over the following few weeks. It was designed to prepare Ben for what to expect before, during, and after a transplant. Over the course of the next ten days, it lived on our kitchen table, available to both of us. I read it with a highlighter in my hand, writing notes and questions and lists in the margins. Each time Ben started to read it, he fell asleep.

CHAPTER 3

Down the Rabbit Hole

March 2020

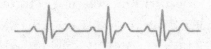

As the second week of March got underway and the first cases of that highly infectious novel virus were identified in New York City, following what everyone hoped was an isolated case in Washington State during January, we both were exhausted. Ben's physical issues were taking up a lot of my bandwidth, and my hospital stay had wiped me out.

Oh . . . and we had moved.

Over the course of the two weekends that bracketed my hospital stay, we relocated around 120 yards from one beloved two-story four-bedroom house to another.

Despite appearing abrupt, the step was actually quite deliberate, taken after much thought and consideration. We'd admired the new place from afar for years: we knew it had great spirit, "good bones," and a splendid location.

It backed immediately onto the park that anchored the whole neighborhood with beautiful trees and a necklace of small saltwater ponds and waterfalls populated with all sorts of critters—an enchanting spot for morning walks or nighttime wildlife "safaris" with the grandchildren. Ben had such an affinity for the park that, despite his medical issues, he had advocated creating and heading up a lakes committee in our community to spotlight the health of the ecosystem and bring in new blood to its operation. Through the winter, even as his powers of concentration deteriorated markedly, somehow the park engaged his imagination and offered him a focal point, a lifeline.

The new house had been designed and built around a dozen years earlier by its only owner, Helene, who had christened it Park Place. When she'd let on just before the holidays that she was downsizing and planning to move in March or April, Ben and I marveled at the timing. Even as we were quite happy and settled where we were, we'd noticed upon our return from Pennsylvania that our front steps, garage stairway, and staircase to the master bedroom were becoming worrisome barriers to his getting around easily. The new house had a wheelchair-accessible entry through the garage and a small elevator to the second floor, two amenities that sounded, based on the anticipated continued progression of Ben's systemic sclerosis and whatever it might do to his heart, like good investments for the future. Finally, Helene's housekeeper, Maria, who'd known and worked in the home since its construction, had agreed to continue to provide much-needed TLC a few afternoons a week.

Ben Reflects

At one point, as I was utterly failing physically and becoming feeble, Sarah told me she was trying to envision our future together as an old couple. "So when we look for our next house," she said, "whatever we do, we're going to look for one that has extra-wide doors and ground-level living."

Then, miraculously, a new house became available. We were trying to set Sarah up there because we thought I was going to die. We settled our affairs, so she had the perfect house in the perfect neighborhood where she could have the best life she could without me.

This house is exactly what we needed. I can drive right into the garage and enter on a wheelchair ramp. I've got the whole first floor to live on. And if I need to be in a recovery suite upstairs, I can wheel myself into the elevator, and up I go.

We'd always done a lot of household projects on our own, but for this relocation we knew not to mess around. We employed movers and solicited help from a team of loving and hardworking friends. While for months to come we would have pictures to hang, home offices to arrange, kitchen cupboards to organize, and books to shelve, thanks to everyone's generous gift of time, the basics were knocked out in just a few days, and we were remarkably well settled, even if every room still had a collection of boxes yet to be emptied. And we'd managed it all just in time for the world to shut down, borders to be sealed, professional sports seasons to be canceled, and schools to close. National orders were issued: Americans should shelter in place for at least two weeks to "flatten the curve" and help prevent the spread of the strange new coronavirus, officially dubbed COVID-19.

But because Ben's sleep issues grew profoundly worse almost immediately, we barely paid attention to the larger world's problems. During the quietest hours of the night, he'd talk in his sleep. In full voice, he would hold extended conversations with himself that could be heard two rooms away: "Yes, two flights of stairs" . . . "We're going to have to discuss that further" . . . "Ow! Ow! Ow!" . . . "Did you manage to get that second IV into my ankle?"

After having fallen out of bed a month earlier and narrowly missing cutting his head open on the bedside table in the process, as soon as we moved, he adopted the couch in the living room as his new "bed" so as to be closer to the floor if he rolled off again. I'd fall asleep in our new first-floor bedroom with the door open, marveling at his one-sided nocturnal conversations . . . on the nights he was calm.

If he wasn't calm, I'd get up and check on him repeatedly, sometimes more than twenty times between midnight and 6:00 a.m. Especially difficult was the week he began using a CPAP device in hopes that it would resolve some of his troubles. It was intended to help keep his breathing airways open and provide a steady flow of oxygen to his system, but not even half awake, he'd tear it off or unsnap the straps once he got to dreaming. Other times, he'd pull away so the air pipe would disconnect from the compressor. At that raspy Darth Vader sound, I'd go out and talk him into putting the whole contraption together again and fasten it back on. If he could stay mostly in a dream state throughout the interaction, he was cooperative; if I had to wake him up, he was not.

Exhaustion so overwhelmed him that in the early hours of one morning, he fell asleep midstride while taking the ten steps back to the couch from the powder room. How I slept through that I have no clue; I only learned about it a few days later.

"What's up with all the ibuprofen?"

"Oh, I tripped in the living room the other night."

"On what?"

"Don't know. I was asleep."

"You mean you were sleepwalking?"

"More like I was awake when I walked into the bathroom and asleep when I walked out."

"So what hurts?"

"My hip."

"Ooh—ouch. Did you hit the coffee table on your way down?"

"I don't think so. It's just that I landed funny and got a bad bruise."

One noontime, he was working on setting up his office, enjoying the view of the park and organizing his desk, when he texted me that he had something that needed to be mailed but couldn't find his roll of postage stamps. I grabbed some from the kitchen drawer and took them upstairs.

"Oh, thanks. Just stick one on this envelope."

I took the envelope, which was addressed but unsealed and empty. "Do you want me to mail it for you?"

"Yes, please."

"Is there supposed to be something in it?"

"Oh. Um. Hang on." He moved a few different piles of paper around on his desk and looked under several others.

"Here it is, and I need to include a check." He turned and gave a form to me. I took the piece of paper, then handed it right back.

"It looks like it needs to be signed and dated at those highlighted spaces."

"Ah. Right." He turned back to his desk and signed it, then stopped. From where I was standing just behind him, I assumed he was rereading it one last time before dating it. But he was taking a long time. Then he started to snore.

"Ben!"

"Oh . . . sorry . . . wait, let me date it."

"Okay. And then I'll just enclose a check with it, if that works for you."

"Yes, please. Thank you. I guess I'll go lie down."

Because he was sleeping so unreliably, he was on three new medications in addition to the CPAP. The impact was confounding.

There were moments in the middle of the day when he'd be talking almost coherently, then say something odd, making it obvious that he was no longer awake but suddenly sound asleep with his eyes wide open. As a passenger in the car, he might abruptly point at something and say "There!" and as the driver, I'd think he was instructing me immediately to change lanes or avoid a road hazard only to realize he was out cold. If we were having a meal together, he might move an empty hand toward his mouth as if he were sipping a drink, and then startle, stop, look at me, pick up his glass, and take a sip for real.

At 4:00 a.m. one Sunday just past the middle of March, I found him sitting on the front stoop with the front door wide open and the porch light blazing. I'm not sure what woke me—perhaps ice cubes hitting the kitchen floor as he filled a cup he was dreaming was in his hand—but by the time I emerged from our bedroom, I could see several of the cubes melting as our ten-year-old black Lab, Savvy—short for Savannah—spirited others away to her bed one at a time, happy to chew on them.

"Ben? Is everything okay? Why are you sitting out here?"

"I'm waiting for the EMTs."

"Excuse me?"

"I need them to help me with my meds. All the pills are in a big pile, turning brown and sticking together."

All Ben's meds—and there were a lot of them—were stored in the medicine cabinet in our bathroom, nowhere near the living-room couch. I wasn't sure, but I didn't think he'd been in there since the previous evening.

The predawn hour was silent, too early even for the birds, and there was no sound of sirens, even though the closest ambulance bay was only a mile away.

"Ben, you need to tell me: Did you really call the EMTs? Do you think you called 911?"

"I don't know. I can't find my phone. But in case I did, we need to stay out here, or at least leave the front door open."

"All right. While we wait, how about I get you a glass of juice?"

"Okay. Maybe I'll come with you and have some breakfast." Any thoughts he had of the EMTs or gooey meds had—*poof!*—disappeared.

I guided him through the house, unnerved by his half-awake state. In the kitchen, he insisted he could prepare his own meal and proceeded to get out a plate, a knife and fork, a tomato, and an unpeeled banana, then wandered onto the back porch as I picked up the last of the ice cubes and toweled the floor dry. When I joined him, I offered to peel the banana, since his manual dexterity had diminished considerably by that point. But he said, "No, thanks. I've got it."

I excused myself, saying I needed to use the bathroom, and went to listen once more for any approaching emergency vehicle. Then I closed the front door and turned off the front porch lights. I returned to the back porch to find him sound asleep, not having eaten a thing. When I woke him, he snapped uncharacteristically, "Okay! Okay! Make me go inside. I'll just eat inside if that's what you want me to do!"

He sat down angrily at the kitchen table and tried unsuccessfully to slice the tomato but kept dozing off. Not wanting him to fall onto the floor, I gently tapped on his shoulder, which only made him angrier. Then he gave up on the tomato and started stabbing at the unpeeled banana, trying to slice it as if it were a piece of meat, repeatedly dozing off but telling me each time I woke him that he was "Fine!" Again he'd assured me that he had the situation under control, "Thank. You. Very. Much."

Not wanting to leave him unattended, finally, somehow, I helped him return to the couch, where he fell back asleep as if he'd been sleeping soundly all night.

James Reflects

I think my mother coped as best she could—with managing details, recording doctors' notes, arranging calendars, and a million other things. When we spoke about Dad in the months before the transplant, it was always with a bit of humor, but we could also tell that she was conveying information that could be hard to hear.

There was some story about Dad making a tomato sandwich in the middle of the night, being angry that the bread wasn't tomatoes or something ridiculous like that. The story superficially rings of humor but simultaneously illustrates just how wrong things were in his head. You could tell Mom was trying to find a balance between letting us know what was going on and not wanting to burden us. I appreciate her finding that balance for herself and for us, her kids.

But there was more. Those ulcers, the ones that had been festering on his ankles since before Thanksgiving, were now infected with pseudomonas and were being treated with IV antibiotics.

Here. In our new home of two weeks.

Which was probably going to prove a roadblock to getting him on the transplant list.

It was a frustrating subject between us. Even though I knew everything else that was going on with Ben medically, he'd never revealed back in October and November of 2019 that this little piece of history was repeating itself, so that by the time he realized the sores weren't going to heal on their own and admitted their existence to me (thank you, ten-year-old boy), they had devastated his skin and become deeply infected. In desperation, I called in a dear friend, Mona, whose nursing background meant Ben might listen to her. Thankfully, she was able to convince him that the infection needed to be investigated and helped him get a prescription to visit a wound clinic several times a week.

The first of those visits to a facility twenty-five miles farther south in the Keys occurred while I was in the hospital, and he reported that things were improving. But apparently, the improvements were too few, because in the interim an IV medication had been prescribed. The prescription included insurance coverage for two nurse visits a week, which meant that the task of administering the twice-daily doses the other dozen times fell to me. As Ben and all our relations know, I am terrible about needles and sera, but fortunately, along with the prescription, he'd received a PICC line—a peripherally inserted central catheter.

Mercifully, it only took a few lessons before I was able to manage the process. Barely. With a lot of deep breathing.

I did, however, order smelling salts from an online pharmacy. Just in case.

That particular morning, having gotten him back to bed after our bizarre interaction about the EMTs, his meds being in a pile, and that strange breakfast, I let him sleep as long as I could. But after preparing everything to do with the IV and not wanting to fall too far behind on the medication schedule, I had no choice; I shook him awake and persuaded him to move to the chair in our bedroom, where we'd set up our own mini clinic, complete with IV pole and all the supplies. He usually dozed once the medicine was flowing, and so he did this time.

Forty minutes later, as I capped off the PICC line, having given him a saline flush, the meds, another saline flush, and heparin, then gathered up and disposed of all the paraphernalia, Ben mumbled, "We probably ought to do my IV now."

In a different time and place, the person I would have gone to for advice and reassurance in the midst of such confusion was Ben; the shoulder I would have leaned on was his.

The reality crushed me.

Late the next morning, I was working through a series of physical therapist–assigned back exercises when I heard a soft thump somewhere upstairs. Curious and a little anxious, I went to explore, finding Ben on his hands and knees in the bathroom next to his office.

He had a goose egg on his forehead, a scrape on his cheek, and a bloody finger. His explanation: he had fallen asleep on the commode.

He'd fallen out of bed at the end of February, hurt his hip a few days previously, and now this, his third fall in as many weeks. That I knew of.

Our lives were collapsing around us, and I had no idea what to do or where to turn. Even during proper real-world waking hours, Ben's fatigue was leading to terrifying disconnects whenever we talked through family business, tried to coordinate calendars, or negotiated as to who'd handle which bills or sign off on paperwork. There was no room for the luxury of thoughtful consideration of our circumstances, for discussion, for problem-solving. I was in panic mode.

If I called a doctor, what would I say? "Ben's becoming a danger to himself" sounded melodramatic, and was I really sure about that? At this point, I was sleep-deprived too, and to my ears, any description of his behavior came across as simultaneously sensational and inadequate. We had become like a pair of frogs in a warm pot of water on the stove: as the heat rose, we became less and less able to jump out and save ourselves. We were being boiled alive.

Ben Reflects

I had become a burden at home. I had awful sleep problems and even started sleepwalking. I was dozing off in the daytime. I couldn't concentrate on anything. It was increasingly difficult to just get around, and I was falling down.

Because my heart wasn't strong enough to pump blood down to my feet, my ankles got infected, wouldn't heal, and we ended up talking about amputation! It was a grim period. I wound up on intravenous antibiotics. And by the time we were in over our heads, it felt like there was no turning back.

I felt really sorry that I was doing this to Sarah and wished I could have been of more help. There she was, putting her life on hold to do something that was not strengthening her in any way. It just got worse and worse. I felt just so frustrated that I couldn't do anything. I was watching her try to fix something that she didn't know how to fix.

Weeks earlier, when we'd returned from the Cleveland Clinic with the transplant book, I'd left it on the kitchen table, but eventually, it migrated to the bench at the foot of our bed. Ben had shown little to no interest, likely because the subject matter was too intense and cut too close to the bone. Having it within easy reach, however, meant I could easily find it, pick it up, read it, and digest it at bedtime or in the middle of the night. And rather than add it to the pile of books on my bedside table, I wanted to keep it where Ben could see it any time he wandered into the room, just in case he found the energy to scan it. It was written so it could be absorbed in short bursts; its stated purpose was to "prepare you for what to expect before, during, and after your heart transplant."

These days, the only things for which Ben was able to muster any energy were puttering about in the garage, deciding where he wanted all those mechanical kinds of things (some still in boxes) to be placed in our new home, and crafting fun plans and projects for the lakes outside our back door.

So it was no real surprise that I was the one picking up the transplant book, studying it, marking paragraphs, and writing questions and comments in the margins.

It covered everything from the most basic information—there was a diagram called "How Your Heart Works," explaining blood flow, coronary arteries, and the heartbeat—to a complete listing of the cardiac transplant team members, including surgeons, cardiologists, coordinators, clinicians, social workers, financial counselors, and others. It began with discussions about heart failure, devices, and medications, then moved through medical history and all the diagnostic tests required in advance, including dental and psychosocial evaluations.

One of the first sentences I highlighted, thinking Ben and I would laugh about it at dinner some night soon, was "Making other major life changes, such as moving . . . is not recommended at this time."

I noticed that the book stressed the need for the patient to stay in the vicinity of the hospital for four to six weeks immediately after the transplant.

Then came a page titled "The Wait":

Acceptance into our program as a heart transplant candidate means the transplant team believes:

- your heart condition is severe enough to warrant this aggressive therapy;
- the transplant surgery will make you feel better, keep you out of the hospital, and prolong your life; and
- there are no conditions that would prevent a successful surgery and recovery.

On the reverse side of that same page, the status rankings for adults waiting for transplant, 1A, 1B, 2, and 7, were explained in devastating detail. The 1A rank was for people who needed mechanical assist devices and intensive intravenous medications in ICU settings and had a life expectancy of less than seven days. At the other end of the spectrum, part of the description of status 7 mentioned a possible reason for the ranking: "A problem may have developed that makes transplantation unwise."

I highlighted "Some people wait only a few days, while others wait for a month or a year or longer." A few pages later, I underlined "The list is based on blood type, body size, UNOS [United Network for Organ Sharing] status, and length of time on the waiting list," and a few pages after that, "If you are planning a trip out of town, please tell the transplant office where you will be and, if applicable, where the closest airport is located."

That might prove important: our son Benjamin was to be married in Nashville in early May, an event I had mentioned during a preliminary interview with one of the transplant surgeons. He hadn't skipped a beat: "If we list you, I will try to be sure you are able to go to your son's wedding, but if a heart becomes available that weekend, you may have to leave the reception before the first dance. Be sure we always know how to reach you."

The paragraph headed "Getting the Call" merited not only my highlighter but also my handwritten circles and arrows to be sure we'd be able to find these crucial instructions instantly.

It concluded with "Once you are called, *do not eat or drink anything* and *keep your telephone line open.* Bring a one-day supply of medications and this transplant notebook with you." In the margin, I added "Hearing aids?" and boxed it in dark ink.

There were descriptions of the cardiac ICU and how long family members could stay with the patient prior to surgery. The process of evaluating the donor heart was delineated. How the patient gets to the OR. Anesthesia details.

And a paragraph headed "Dry Run," which read, "There is always a possibility that the donor heart is not functioning properly, or the donor may become too unstable to continue with transplant. The surgeon will inform you of this event as soon as they are aware of the situation. Please do not be too disappointed if this happens."

After reading that, I touched based with college roommate Jon to ask, "How often does it turn out to be a dry run?"

"Maybe one time in ten."

The various methods of surgery were explained, along with post-op recovery and the fact that, once the patient moves from the ICU to the nursing unit, it is the patient's responsibility to ask for pain medication.

I dog-eared the page that listed the post-transplant symptoms of infection requiring immediate contact with a health-care provider. A couple of pages later, a paragraph that sounded COVID-inspired merited yellow highlighter: *Family and friends should clean their hands with soap and water or an alcohol-based hand rub before and after visiting you. If you do not see them clean their hands, please ask them to do so.*

There were dietary suggestions and wound care instructions and cautions: Do not drive a car for six weeks after your surgery. Do not lift anything over 10–20 pounds for six weeks. Do not go into crowded places for the first three months. Do not work in or visit any form of construction site.

There was also a chart: "How to know if your incision is infected." Plus a schedule of postsurgical biopsies. Symptoms of rejection. Reminders about the importance of taking medications at the correct time each day.

When I read "Call your doctor if your sternum (breastbone) feels like it moves or it pops or cracks with movement," I reached for my smelling salts.

As the last week of March began, we were eager to grab hold, even for just five minutes, of some semblance of our former "normal" lives, despite the fact that the broader world's concept of normal had been turned upside down by the COVID-19 global health emergency. In the United States, the Centers for Disease Control and Prevention had recently confirmed the first case in an American who had neither traveled abroad nor knowingly come in contact with an already infected person. A national task force was established.

In his declaration of a national emergency a few days earlier, the president had issued guidelines: for thirty days, everyone was to limit discretionary travel and avoid gatherings of more than ten people in order to slow the spread.

On day 12 or 13 of the pandemic, we were in our new garage when my phone pinged with a text message just as Ben and I were about to pretend for a little while that, somehow, we could time-travel back to what our lives had been like three years earlier.

That afternoon, Ben had asked, "Wanna go tour the park with me? Look at the ponds, check the waterfalls, see some birds, count some fish, maybe stay out long enough to watch the sun set over Card Sound and spy a dolphin or two?" The western views over the water toward the Everglades could be breathtaking.

I'd jumped up from my desk, turned the knob on the Crock-Pot to Warm, grabbed some soft drinks and sleeves to keep them cold, and followed him as he limped to the golf cart.

In the garage, I checked my phone. "This is odd—it's a Connecticut area code with a weird photo."

I held the phone out so Ben could see it. "Can you tell what this is a photo of? Is it a snake, maybe? Say, under a table?"

"It is. It's a black racer." His lucidity in the wake of so many incoherent episodes over the previous several weeks freaked me out. He snapped to attention, a man on a mission.

"Text back and ask where I need to be; I'll grab a net. Can you go grab a pillowcase?"

As he limped to the cupboard on the other side of the garage and I went to find a pillowcase, I dictated a reply: "Sorry, I'm not recognizing this phone number, but Ben is really excited about the snake. He'd be thrilled to come get it right now. Where do you need him?"

The reply came: "This is Alfredo. Your husband asked me to call when we see one of these."

Alfredo was the assistant manager of the fishing club right around the corner, and he lived next door to our old house.

I responded, "Are you at work? Or home?"

"Work. Please ask him to come to the clubhouse, front entrance."

"On our way!"

Because of the COVID guidelines in place following the president's directive, the whole country was living as if every individual had received a heart transplant—hypervigilant about cleanliness and potential exposure to germs. Whether face masks might be effective was still up for debate, but there weren't enough of them for medical personnel, so everyone had been asked to refrain from hoarding them. Desperate people began stockpiling toilet paper instead.

In the meantime, no one could determine who among us might be carrying the virus but not yet showing symptoms. Even the president, who had declared early on that it would go away quickly, had finally come around to acknowledging, "This is bad," predicting that the crisis could last "into July, or August, or longer."

In our neighborhood, that meant the clubhouse had been shut down immediately except for take-out meals, so it was strange to arrive and find the French doors at the front entrance wide open. Stranger still to find Alfredo and seven staff members waiting in the long, narrow lobby and a thirty-inch black snake under the table just inside the doors, coiled up tightly as far back against the wall as it could get.

As we entered, everyone shifted according to some strange COVID choreography: one person would move, then all the others automatically adjusted to maintain their separate spaces.

Ben took charge.

"Alfredo, Paul, Shawn—the three of you block the front doorway in case it heads that way. Robert, John, and Danny, you three do the same with the double doors to the living room."

Then, as he gingerly got in position to lie down on the limestone floor, he continued, "Sarah and Jim [yes, that Jim—the security guard who'd been present when Ben caught the python], grab the cushions from that chair and help me lie down, then Sarah, be ready with the pillowcase. Christian, slowly extend this net behind the snake from over there. I'm thinking I should be able to grab it, but I may miss the first time. Everybody ready?"

Everyone nodded.

"Here goes!"

Then *whoop!* Ben darted his hand in and grasped the snake just behind its head as it whipped and wound around his arm.

"Is that snake poop?"

"Is that blood?"

"Do we need bandages?"

"Mr. Cart, are you okay?"

It was like Christmas all over again, and Ben wasn't paying attention to anything except the snake, so I answered all four questions: "Yes, yes, yes, and yes."

Pandemic mode dictated the rest; everyone continued to maintain their distance, taking turns using the hand sanitizer that was on the table. Alfredo disappeared momentarily, then reappeared with antiseptic and bandages. Somehow, Paul had anticipated how the adventure might go and so had been properly equipped with paper towels and all-purpose cleanser.

And Ben was happily giving a science lesson.

"Black racers are nonvenomous. This is a good-size one. They always poop like that when you pick them up. Yes, it bit me, but that was just in fear and self-defense, and it doesn't hurt.

"Here: touch its skin; feel its scales. It's not slimy.

"Can you tell how strong it is? It's flicking its tongue like that because that's how it smells and tries to figure out what's going on and whether there's prey around.

"It's a perfect size to keep as a pet for a couple weeks; I'll set it up in a terrarium in my office, and we'll feed it lizards." Referencing a favorite film franchise, he concluded, "I think I'll name it John Wick."

CHAPTER 4

Do Not Go Gentle into That Good Night

March 27—March 30, 2020

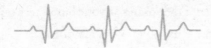

We will never know if our farewell would have been different if we'd had any idea what was in store. As it was, our parting came about quickly—the way you're supposed to pull off a Band-Aid.

The landline rang late on a Friday afternoon. I happened to answer it in the kitchen. It was Carlos, calling to say he was "concerned about Ben's most recent blood work."

"Wow! That was fast!"

He hesitated, then asked, "What do you mean?"

"Are you talking about the blood draw this afternoon?"

"He had blood drawn this afternoon?"

"Uh . . . yes. For the infectious-disease doctor, to see if the IV antibiotics are helping with that pseudomonas infection in his ankles."

"The results I'm looking at are from Monday. There are some screwy numbers here."

The only words I comprehended well enough to latch onto as Carlos continued were "His salts are low."

"What's that number?"

"It's 121."

We'd learned that the normal range for salt was between 135 and 145 when Ben's father's salts had been elevated during the final months of his life, five years earlier, and again when Ben's numbers had been low two years previously. "Oh. Crap. Well, that explains a thing or two."

"How do you mean?"

"He's been, um, easily confused."

"Well, he would be."

At this point, Ben picked up the extension in his office and asked, "Is this for me?"

"Hey there, Ben. I'm looking at your blood test results—"

"Oh, hi, Carlos. Wow—you guys are quick!"

"Nope: not from today; from Monday. There are numbers here that are screwy—low salts and bad kidney numbers."

"How so?"

"I think you should be checked out."

"Um. Well. Okay. If you're on call this weekend, I can come see you in the morning. Pee in a cup, let you draw some more blood, whatever you need."

"No. You need to see somebody tonight."

"You mean I need to go to the emergency room?"

"I'm not sure; I think maybe you should go all the way to the clinic as soon as possible. Let me call your cardiologist and get back to you."

"Now?"

"Yeah. I'll call you right back."

Having hung up, I stopped by our bedroom to grab a couple of things before apprehensively climbing the stairs to join Ben in his office, wait for Carlos's call, and talk through what items Ben might want in his go bag. Between his having to be "dried out" in Hartford Hospital the previous summer and my four nights in Miami just a few weeks previously, we had plenty of experience on that score.

As I walked in, Ben was already on his cell phone to Lamar, the driver who had been handling Ben's transportation needs when I was unavailable. Now Carlos was suggesting that Ben might have to get to the Cleveland Clinic, seventy miles away, on a Friday evening—ASAP.

Ben knew he didn't want me to drive, because except for short jaunts, I hadn't been behind the wheel of a car since being discharged, and he didn't want to go by ambulance, so if Lamar were available and willing . . . Fortunately, he was on both counts. He promised Ben he could be at our door within half an hour if need be.

I'd entered Ben's office with a bag and a list. "So. I've grabbed your iPad, its charger, your phone charger, your CPAP, your hearing aids' dock and cord, a notepad, and a pen. Anything else? A change of clothes?"

"My license and insurance card plus an extension cord, please. My wallet should stay here. I really don't want the CPAP, but yeah, maybe. No clothes. If they keep me, they'll put me in a gown, and I can wear these clothes there and back."

The landline rang, and I picked it up; it was Carlos. "I got through to Dr. Bush, and he agrees. Ben needs to get to the clinic tonight. He should go to the emergency-room entrance; they'll be expecting him."

"All right. Ben got a hold of a driver while we were waiting to hear back from you. He can be here in twenty-five minutes, which puts Ben at the clinic around 8:00 p.m. Do you think he'll have to spend the night? Or should the driver plan to wait for him?"

Hearing me, Ben was already dialing Lamar to finalize arrangements even as Carlos continued. "Sarah, based on his numbers, I think they're going to have to admit him; I think he's going to be there for a while."

"But with this virus going around? Will he be safe there? I feel like you're asking us to send him into the belly of the beast."

"It might be the safest place for him—certainly safer than keeping him home when he's flunked his blood work this badly. They know him and his situation; despite the risks, it's what needs to happen."

The front door was open and the porch lights were on when Lamar pulled up twenty-five minutes later in a sleek black Suburban. Savvy was all wiggles and wags: Lamar's arrivals had become a highlight for her. He always greeted her with a tummy rub.

Although I'd been reserved about touching Ben ever since my own hospital stay in case I'd picked up any germs that had yet to manifest themselves, I quietly laid my hands on his shoulders and gave him a kiss on the cheek before he turned to give Lamar the go bag and the cane he and Lamar had picked up a few days earlier on one of their roundtrips to the wound clinic. Ben said he found it helpful for his bruised hip.

As Lamar placed those items in the back of his Suburban, Ben, always the optimist, said, "Here I go, Mama Cart. They'll fix whatever this is, and maybe while I'm there, we'll knock out the last few procedures that need to get done so they can get me on 'the list,' and then I'll be on my way back to you, and the wait can begin."

"On my way back to you" was a phrase we frequently used whenever one of us was looking for the other after a day's meetings or errands. In text speak, we had come to abbreviate it as OMWB2U.

Lamar helped Ben climb into the back seat and closed the door.

Part of me was watching this from someplace far, far away. My stomach was tight. I forced a smile.

Ben lowered his window as Lamar walked around to settle into the driver's seat. "My phone's fully charged; I'll keep you posted. Get some sleep."

"I'm going to hold off on reaching out to the boys and your sister. But your mother will want to hear your voice."

"I'll give her a call from the car."

"I love you."

"I love you too."

The SUV pulled away. Savvy and I stood in the driveway; she wagged her tail, and I waved until the car was out of sight. Then she and I turned and went into the new house. I closed the front door and locked it, flicked the porch lights off, then turned around to look at the hallway, staircase, living room, and, just around the corner, the kitchen and dining room with the elevator beyond. It was eerily quiet. Moving boxes yet to be unpacked were visible in every direction. I was determined not to cry and would simply take things an hour at a time until he got home.

Now it was my turn to have sleep issues.

I lay awake examining the ceiling of our new bedroom until sometime after a 3:30 a.m. unpunctuated text from Ben arrived: "I woke private room I see you first breakfast at eight talk to you then."

Having finally heard from him, initially I focused on the "eight talk to you then" part, knowing he'd explain the late-night nonsense in the morning.

I felt like I could breathe for the first time since the car had pulled away, perhaps even roll over, punch the pillow into just the right shape, pull up the covers, close my eyes, and relax . . . relax . . . relax . . .

I could even hear Savvy finally settle down as she sensed my relief.

"I see you."

Dammit. Now it made sense.

It had taken so long to get him a room because they'd determined that he needed to be in the *ICU.*

When we talked on Saturday morning, Ben reported that yes, he was in a private room in the ICU, but that was great (despite the 5:00 a.m. sponge bath) because the doctors were all over the concept of getting him onto the transplant list. That meant they were treating his infected ankles aggressively with two antibiotics and planning, at long last, to schedule a colonoscopy.

He also shared his surprise—because he had slept through it—that a cardiologist had visited him in the ER, which the nurses pointed out was highly unusual. He wasn't overwhelmingly coherent, but by the time we spoke again that evening, he sounded more like himself. I attributed the improvement to rehydration and meds.

A couple of hours later, I called the hospital to ask about visiting hours and learned to my bitter disappointment that it didn't matter whether he was in the ICU or on a regular floor: he wasn't allowed to have visitors.

The rule didn't just apply to friends. It meant no one. No family. No *me*.

Due to COVID, and out of an abundance of caution, the hospital's newly established protocol was no visitors at all. It shouldn't have been a surprise.

I'd noted in my journal just a week earlier: "As half the population of the US has been ordered to shelter in place, we have not yet begun to see the level of destruction COVID-19 will wreak in the next 45 days (an oft-cited time frame of approximately when we'll BEGIN to get an idea of how long this pandemic might go on. Some estimates are 'waves' continuing for more than 18 months.)"

Well, okay then.

Ben was just going to have to be a model patient for a few days, let them fix whatever was wrong so those blood numbers could come back under control, make good progress on the ankle infection, undergo a colonoscopy, then finally get back on track and on "the list" and return home for "the wait."

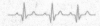

I had a whole weekend ahead of me. I spent that first day "playing busy"—keeping moving, unpacking, sorting, folding, putting things away, walking in circles while trying to make decisions about what to put where.

I also had a to-do list that had been growing over the past several weeks: articles to draft for our local Florida weekly newspaper and for a quarterly newsletter in the Poconos, thank-you notes to write, birthdays and anniversaries to acknowledge. Late that afternoon, I contacted each of our boys and our siblings, plus his mother, my father and stepmother, and a small group of our oldest and closest friends to share what little I knew about what was going on.

And I tried to focus on the fact that, after several challenging months, Ben's hospitalization for a few days might prove a miracle in its own right.

The reality was, I had a lot to be thankful for.

The weather had been gorgeous. My physical therapist had a sixth sense about how best to facilitate strengthening my back and thus aid my complete recovery, and as the coronavirus was gaining momentum, people from all parts of our lives, aware that Ben had been having a tough couple of years, had been wonderfully generous about calling, texting, emailing, and reaching out to see how he and I were faring in light of the international health situation. My usual answer had been that there wasn't much to tell them: "The larder's full; Ben sleeps (restlessly) a lot; but when he's awake, his attitude is good."

But as COVID garnered more attention and whole countries were going into lockdown, I'd been thinking we needed a plan, especially since the virus would limit the options to improve Ben's health. Those limitations terrified me, but if we were going to have to shelter in place for several weeks, perhaps it would be an opportunity for Ben to completely rid himself of the pseudomonas, develop better sleep habits, and build up whatever strength he could—especially if we could clear up his ankle issues, because then, maybe, depending on COVID restrictions, he could get some exercise in the pool over at the neighborhood clubhouse.

And now the hospital was taking care of him, so I had time to lay in supplies and prepare for his homecoming.

These days apart would also be a good test of how well I'd absorbed the content of dozens of conversations Ben and I had had on all sorts of topics since his initial autoimmune diagnosis. We'd come to agree, sort of jokingly, that I was "working on getting a PhD" in our household accounts, general finances, insurance, taxes, and more. The "curriculum" had been challenging on several levels, from discussions of the most sensitive subjects ("If you die, what do I do when . . .") to frequently frustrating exchanges at cross-purposes. I might walk into his office wanting the simplest answer about where to file a form, and he'd launch into a discourse on "cost basis" or borrowing against life insurance or what expenses could be paid from our health savings account and when we'd be eligible to make another deposit into it.

For long periods, knowing he might go off on such lengthy (and at first confusing) tangents, I would avoid asking even the simplest questions. Eventually, however, one afternoon in a tangent-inspired snit, I hit upon a comparison that came to serve as useful shorthand.

"Pretend that for some reason we cannot imagine, I suddenly find myself transported to the middle of a town in Russia with only the clothes on my back. It's cold, and I'm hungry. I don't know where I'm going to spend the night, and I don't speak any Russian. When a local approaches to help, the first thing I want is a jacket, so there's some sign language to that effect, then something to eat, which means more sign language, and finally, some shelter. I'm not ready to learn how to speak Russian, much less sit still for a lesson on Russian grammar.

"My point here is that I have just arrived in your village needing a simple jacket, not a grammar lesson."

After that fit of pique, although the curriculum was occasionally taxing, sticking to the syllabus and asking questions became a lot easier.

"Hey, Ben, how often does this payment have to be made?"

"That? Well, back in Ohio, we always handled it by—"

"I don't have time for a grammar lesson."

"That gets paid every three months. It's paperless; the statement comes to my email address."

"Thank you."

Eventually, I began to get the hang of his various systems, and occasionally, I'd even ask for a "Russian lesson." But too, there were questions that had nothing to do with filing systems and payment schedules. Improbably, some of the toughest questions, the ones that began with "what if" and "when," inspired answers that led to a deeper understanding of him, me, us, and the world we'd built together, even as they diminished my supply of Kleenex.

So I asked questions and took notes and finally drafted a cheat-sheet glossary of sorts full of how-to information. It categorized tasks that needed daily, weekly, monthly, and annual attention. It listed which accounts were on autopay; outlined the seasonal closing and opening procedures for the Poconos cabin and the house in the Keys; identified whom to call among long lists of various vendors and contractors when something went awry; broke down all our various insurance policies (auto, health, homeowners, life, and so on); and included an explanation of COBRA as well as a chart showing when I'd have to look into Medicare.

His being away would be a good test run for me and the cheat sheet. Besides, if a question came up, we could talk about it on the phone.

Still. It was only Saturday. I was happy to avoid his desk for a little longer. Maybe it could even wait until he came home.

On Sunday, Ben reported that the doctors had a few additional procedures on their to-do list, so he was going to remain a guest of the clinic for a few days more. I shared the news of his situation with a few more friends via email and then realized that—*oops!*—it was time for me to play herpetologist and free John Wick. Although I was willing to do a lot on Ben's behalf, capturing anoles and toads and other small critters and insects to feed a black racer just wasn't going to happen.

By Sunday night, I finally recognized and trusted that this was an opportunity for me to get some real sleep. Hello, Tylenol PM! I'd avoided taking any while Ben was home because it hindered my ability to doze with one eye open.

First thing Monday morning, I reviewed what remained on my to-do list in a funk. Over the course of one weekend, I had pretty much burned through my whole reserve of "productive procrastination" feel-good activities. Not a single interesting task remained. Nothing glowed with the promise of becoming an obvious accomplishment. It was all just unsexy stuff that oughta get done, and I knew I'd eventually be grateful for having done it, but immediate motivation was sorely lacking. Settling into the new house and making it feel like ours held less than zero appeal without Ben to help or offer opinions or even disagree with the choices I might make about where to unroll a rug, place a piece of furniture, or hang a picture.

I needed structure to get through this pandemic, and with Ben in the hospital, as a distraction, I typed a to-do list into the Notes app on my phone.

It was a start—a semblance of a routine from which to deviate. In the days to come, it would evolve to include new feel-good accomplishments, from "Call nurses' station" and "Meditate" to "Empty moving boxes in [such and such room] and put stuff away."

It probably should have included "Go watch the sunset," but while I was happy to look west over the water during the day, to do so in the evening, something Ben and I had been doing together ever since we moved into the neighborhood six years earlier, demanded a bravado I just wasn't able to muster.

Around noon on that first Monday without Ben, I answered a phone call from the clinic's cath lab.

"Is this Mrs. Cart?"

It was an interventional radiologist. He introduced himself and explained that we were on speakerphone and that there was a nurse there to serve as witness to our conversation, which would have to suffice because I couldn't be present at the hospital.

"Can you tell me your husband's full name and date of birth?"

My correct answers were necessary before they could ask for my consent, he said. "Oh? For a colonoscopy?"

"Uh, no. The doctors would like to do a right heart catheterization and a liver biopsy via your husband's jugular, after which he will be moved to the medical ICU."

There was also discussion of inserting a Swan-Ganz catheter in his pulmonary artery. I felt an urge to find my smelling salts. This didn't sound like a colonoscopy was going to happen anytime soon or that the doctors were thinking of sending Ben home in a few days.

I asked a few questions, then gave my consent and watched the clock until they called to say things had gone well.

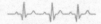

As a result of the procedures, Ben was dopey and out of touch all afternoon, but much to my relief and surprise, that night he dialed into a Zoom call arranged by Pete, the veterinary pathologist college roommate who had served as best man at our wedding, and his wife, Jillian. Considering that Ben had never been on a Zoom call before (and maybe hadn't even heard of it until that day), I was thrilled—not only that he was organized enough to be on it but also that he was so coherent and chipper.

As we ended the call, Pete closed with a signature line of affirmation he'd adopted around ten years earlier and often used on himself, to the amusement of all of us who love him. The original version, spoken when he'd accomplished something of personal import, no matter how small or large, is "Way to go, me!"

That night, he raised our spirits with "Way to go, you!"

CHAPTER 5

Adulting

March 31, 2020—April 9, 2020

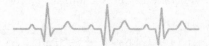

After my Tuesday morning shower, I resolved to be a grown-up and tackle the paperwork on Ben's desk. I poured a cup of coffee, went to sit in his office, and tried to make some sense of the piles of folders, different-size notepads, and odd scraps of paper.

Then Dr. Bush called to bring me up to date.

He reported that Ben had one issue in particular delaying any consideration of listing him for transplant, and to my surprise, the lack of a colonoscopy wasn't it. The infected ankles, while worrisome, weren't it, either. Rather, it was the severe Raynaud's.

Because Raynaud's restricts circulation to the extremities, and the transplant post-op medications can put extremities at risk, Ben could lose anything from toes and fingers to a leg or forearm to amputation. Fortunately, the team hadn't decided yay or nay yet. All I could muster in response was that while I wasn't sure what Ben would say, my point of view was that I'd rather have him back missing a limb than not have him at all.

As for Ben's liver biopsy, Dr. Bush explained that it had been necessary because of the "failed blood work" but had gone well, terming it "a box to be checked." Another box would be a colonoscopy, if they could get him one. Ironically, as unpleasant as colonoscopies are, they are considered elective, and, due to COVID, no elective surgeries were allowed.

Dr. Bush asked if I had any questions. Later, I'd come up with dozens, but at that moment, I had only one: When might I be able to visit?

"Sorry, but there aren't any exceptions to the COVID protocol of no visitors right now."

And, he acknowledged, "It doesn't sound like those restrictions will be lifted in the near future."

Thankfully, Ben had his phone and his iPad so he and I could Face-Time, but for now I had to learn my way around his desk.

I spent more than four hours there on Tuesday and invested another two first thing on Wednesday, finding it sobering and a bit terrifying to realize how disoriented he had been for so long. There were several items not entered into the check register. There were bills that were past due buried deep in the folder; such items were supposed to be placed in chronological order with the most pressing on top so they'd get handled in a timely fashion. Some bills were overpaid; others were underpaid. I also found weeks-old emails that ought to have been met with prompt responses upon receipt.

Ben Reflects

As my world got smaller, and as I had diminishing contact with everyone and everything I was familiar with, I found myself less able to focus on daily life. Everything but my immediate physical needs dropped off my radar. I didn't have the time or the bandwidth to be deep and thoughtful about anything.

None of this should have been news to me. A couple of weeks earlier, I had stumbled across the fact that our most recent credit card bill hadn't been paid. Ben had intended to do so online and had done everything except hit the Submit button, but the issues I was finding now were on a completely different scale.

After a break and needing to buck myself up for another run at it, I vowed that each day, until I felt I knew my way around and was caught up, I would set a timer for one hour. If there was still stuff needing attention at that point, it would just have to wait.

Although Ben and I had been speaking and texting numerous times a day, except after his Monday procedures, I didn't mention the issues at his desk, and while I expressed intense disappointment at the COVID restrictions and the possible Raynaud's glitch, he remained upbeat. He was optimistic that not only would the Raynaud's problem work itself out, the transplant team would also put him on "the list" any minute now, and then he'd be "OMWB2U, baby!" He'd be able to come home, and we'd be able to wait together. In the meantime, he was pleased that the doctors had him doing some physical therapy, and the IV antibiotics and diuretics were flowing into him constantly, so he was hopeful that the pseudomonas infection in his ankles was finally going to be resolved.

Then in the middle of the night, despite the Tylenol PM, I woke with a start. Having experienced our parents' hospitalizations in recent years, I realized that Ben might not simply get "discharged to home." In fact, there might be a stay in a rehab facility first. Thinking about what I'd found sitting at his desk, I wondered if there was such a thing as rehab for executive function. And would rehab let me visit? Or were there going to be COVID restrictions there too?

The next morning, I received a cheery phone call from Ben's mother, who lived with 24-7 care in a Poconos cabin a quarter mile from ours. Knowing I was still recovering from my own hospital stay, she offered to pay for a car that would take me to visit him. I thanked her for the lovely thought but then had to explain that as much as I missed him and was desperate to see him, he couldn't have visitors in the ICU, and with the

pandemic, even if he were on a regular floor, I wouldn't dare risk exposing him or myself or others to the virus.

Later in the week, I admitted to my own physical therapist with
some concern and confusion that my back felt "fragile," similar to, but
only fractionally, the way it felt the day it had given out a month earlier.
Christine knew about Ben's situation and that I'd been on my own. In her
wisdom, she asked quietly, "So how did you spend your day yesterday?"

"I did the exercises you've given me. Got out for a couple decent
walks. Although I unpacked a moving box or two, I didn't do any
heavy lifting."

She also knew about my volunteer activities and work for our community's weekly paper, which meant time spent at my computer, so she
persisted. "How about sitting at your desk?"

"Ah. Well, I didn't sit at mine much, but I told myself I was going to
sit at Ben's for an hour, and it ended up being three and a half."

"Bingo!" She smiled as if she'd known that would be the answer,
then continued: "You can't do that anymore. You need to get up and
stretch at least every twenty minutes."

I was stunned at how quickly she identified the problem.

Speaking of interesting problems, I'd also noticed over the previous forty-eight hours that both Savvy and I were spending a lot of time
scratching. I hadn't given it much thought, but once the mystery of my
back pain was solved, there was space in my head to consider the mystery
of the scratching. Phooey.

We had fleas.

Fortunately, when I called the vet, she told me that she had on hand
oral medications and topical treatments for Savvy. Thank goodness they
started working in less than an hour after I picked them up, so the
pests stopped biting her immediately. And Maria was happy to get busy
with a deep-cleaning project. Plus, the exterminator agreed to come first
thing the next day, and he scheduled a follow-up visit in a couple of
weeks to address the next hatch. Unfortunately, though, fleas find me
as tasty as they find the dog, and despite slathering myself with insect

repellent, I was going to be at their mercy until the exterminator's solutions kicked in.

It had been a long time since I'd had to deal with such pests, and as Maria and I washed the covers on the dog beds and all our bed linens, I had to laugh at the realization that they come in waves, kind of like a pandemic. And I was grateful that Ben wasn't home to be subjected to the upheaval, although I hoped he'd be home by the time the exterminator returned.

Thursday night, as Ben and I spoke on the phone and reflected on his full week at the clinic, we agreed that his days were long and, sometimes, productive. His liver biopsy results had come back clean, just as the doctors expected, which was a good thing, showing that the issues with his blood work appeared to be directly related to congestive heart failure. He was pleased to be getting physical therapy, including assistance for the swollen fingers that were compromising his manual dexterity, and hopeful that it would help with his "activities of daily living" difficulties so he would be able to function better at home.

Regarding the physical therapy, however, he admitted, "It's a bit unnerving to have to use a walker."

"Wait—what?"

"My hip still hurts from that fall last week; the walker helps."

Even so, he was grumpy about the fact that the wound team, which had been scheduled to evaluate the progress on his ankles and change his dressings, hadn't gotten to him the day before. At least he was getting the IV antibiotics, though, and his night nurse, Saul, took a stab at giving him new bandages.

Too, he'd been hoping for a decision from the transplant team. Word had been that they would discuss and consider his case at their Thursday meeting.

"Have you heard anything from them?" he asked.

"Not since Dr. Bush called me on Monday."

I tried to explain where things stood with regard to COVID-19—that the governor had finally issued a "safer at home" directive, but the exemptions were curious: folks couldn't visit loved ones in the hospital, but gun shops, liquor stores, and religious gatherings were all included on the "essentials" list and were able to stay open.

At least that got Ben to laugh. "Maybe it's the meds they have me on, but those exemptions sound crazy."

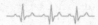

I'd made it to Friday; *we'd* made it to Friday.

Numerous times since mid-March, Elyse, a friend from around the corner, had forwarded a link to me for a free 21-Day Meditation Experience offered by Oprah Winfrey and Deepak Chopra. The celebrity icons had put the series of online videos out there in the world, free, to help people cope with the uncertainties of the pandemic—from being ill to losing a loved one, losing a job, or facing the simply overwhelming prospect of sheltering in place without knowing when all "this" was going to end.

What with the chaos of administering Ben's at-home IV antibiotics, then adjusting to his being in the hospital and learning my way around his desk, I hadn't worked my way back to those emails or the link yet. But whenever I saw Elyse out and about, she kept pushing, gently, and first thing Friday morning, I finally signed on and went through the day 1 offering. After listening to the introductions and meditating with the provided soundtrack for twenty blissful minutes, I came away with the day's three mantras:

"The power of hope is real."

"Hope is my source of strength."

"I am pure potentiality."

Two hours later, the phone rang. It was as if the universe had heard me. Dr. Viviana Navas, from the transplant team, was on the other end, and Ben was there with her. She was calling from his room, and she wanted to share some news.

He was going on "the list." Ben and I both cried.

We then had a Zoom session with all four of our boys that night. What a gift it was to see and laugh with all of them.

I also sent out a mass email to family, friends, and neighbors—current and past, near and far, north and south, high school and college—which resulted in my receiving dozens of beautiful messages of love and support and prayers. Even as the coronavirus pandemic was turning the whole world on its head, we had an amazing number of blessings to count.

Way to go, us.

Friday, April 3
He's going on the list

Hi, all—

The doctors discussed Ben's case this morning.

There is one bureaucratic bit that needs to happen: insurance has said previously that a heart transplant for Ben will be covered 100%; now they need to say it officially.

And on Monday the doctors plan to insert a Swan-Ganz balloon pump to help his heart function. Dr. Navas, who gave us the news this morning, expects he will stay in the hospital until a donor is found.

So once the insurance confirmation is in, Ben will be on the heart transplant list!! A good and important step in the right direction; counting blessings.

xoxoxo SAC

I slept well that night without any pharmaceutical assistance. Which was a good thing, because it would be a while before that could happen again.

Saturday stretched out ahead of me, another mindlessly long day with a to-do list that just couldn't seem to get completed (at least not sensibly). While there were texts, emails, and phone calls from family and friends to answer, and warm wishes and earnest prayers to be acknowledged, I was nonplussed and stalled out by the idea that he'd be in the hospital for at least a few more weeks, and because the coronavirus situation only appeared to be getting worse, I wouldn't see him.

It didn't help that Ben didn't seem to hear the doctor say that he would be staying at CCF until a donor was found. Our conversations were becoming noticeably hit-and-miss: depending on how well he slept the night before and what medication he was on, he was either wonderfully focused and coherent or a mess of slurred speech and nonsensical non sequiturs ("Oh, did I say that out loud? Sorry—I think I was having an imaginary conversation").

Staring out the front door, I realized that the next day was Palm Sunday and remembered that someone had suggested a safe way to honor the holiday: display palm fronds where friends and neighbors could see them. Soon two perfect ones were propped on either side of the entryway.

The holiday was not on Ben's radar; at 2:00 a.m. Sunday, he texted me with some banking advice regarding items already handled. Then, after being busy in the middle of the night, he was also busy midafternoon. When I called, his nurse informed me that he had been coherent enough to provide his own consent for the next morning's insertion of the Swan-Ganz balloon pump, having discussed it with various members of the team. The doctors, including Jon, via long distance, had assured him that it was his best (read "only") option at this point. The device would officially confirm his list status as a 2, and if he were on it for more than thirty days, his status would rise to 1B; that change could also happen sooner if he required continuous treatment with certain IV medications. In a weak moment, I went online and read lots of statistics regarding how quickly a transplant might follow.

As dawn broke on Monday, I logged on for day 4 of Oprah and Deepak's experience and meditated on the power of hope and radiating confidence and strength. I envisioned the hospital in a cone of light descending from the broad universe and called forth a multitude of

angels, every friend and loved one we'd lost over the years—Ben's father
and grandparents and aunt, my mother and brother, my brother-in-law
and stepbrother, a couple of Ben's best friends from high school, and
countless others. I imagined their energy as focused radiance and asked
them to keep Ben, and his doctors and nurses, safe and strong, COVID-
free, and ready for a miracle. I also pictured Lamar's black Suburban
pulling up to the house, the rear passenger door opening, and Ben arriving home, emerging to enthusiastic wiggles and wags from Savvy and
grateful tears from me.

Then I worked to distraction at his desk and mine, only to learn
that his morning procedure had been postponed until midafternoon
and he'd been sleeping all day. Yet because sometimes I find mindless
procrastination to be the most productive of all activities, I got lots
done: the plumber fixed the drippy sink in the bathroom, the severed
Invisible Fence wire got repaired (by me, thanks to some over-the-phone
tutoring from the tech—"No house calls because of COVID"), and the
electrician agreed to come the following week to talk me through some
weird issues with the exterior lights. Also, the CPA promised he'd let
me know what needed to happen with our 2020 tax returns as well as
some other bureaucratic details to do with the IRS, and the pest-control
guy acknowledged the news that the fleas remained an issue. I sucked it
up and canceled the reservations for our Nashville Airbnb for the early
May wedding of our son Benjamin and his fiancée, Anna, since they'd
decided to postpone the celebration for at least a year, marveling at the
reality that, if the wedding were to happen as planned, the father of the
groom wouldn't have been able to attend—this way, there was a chance,
however slim, that Ben would be present at the celebration. Finally, I
paid our neighborhood-association bill and Ben's last outstanding medical bill, which I'd found tucked away in the wrong file.

All of which was simply to say:

Way to go, me. Let's go, us.

Hang in, Ben.

I had no choice but to believe there were miracles out there just waiting for us to embrace them.

Tuesday brought a cluster of communications challenges. Ben had developed some sort of tremor in his hands that compromised his ability to put in his hearing aids as well as his ability to hold his cell phone. Meanwhile, word came from Petrox of another bookkeeping error Ben had made, this time affecting our COBRA coverage. The error mattered, because although Ben had officially retired on disability, my understanding was that COBRA would be our insurance carrier for at least a year—if what Ben had "taught" me in one of those Russian lessons was correct.

When I tried to explain the situation to him, he struggled mightily to comprehend. To make matters worse, we kept getting disconnected when he'd try to switch between his hearing aids and speakerphone. In theory, by the eighth and final call, he understood the issue, and also in theory, I had resolved it, but I was going to have to wait for the Petrox bookkeeper to confirm that.

And, terrifyingly, in the midst of all those calls (interrupted by breaks that lasted anywhere from thirty seconds to thirty minutes), he sent a text: "I'm on my way."

Tap-tap-tap: "You're on your way where?" No response.

I scrambled to reach his nurse. When I got through, I told her that Ben had sent a bizarre message; was everything okay? While she went to check on him, my head was *all* over the place regarding the meaning of "On my way." To where? To a new room? Another test? The OR? My pulse was racing.

Dammit!

This business of being apart, being unable to communicate clearly, being dependent upon the kindness of strangers for basic information, spending countless minutes on hold nearly every time I tried to track down the latest information about what was going on, who had seen him, what his numbers were and what they meant, advocating on his behalf if I felt something needed to happen but not knowing what I would have been able to glean if I could just *visit* him—it was driving me mad.

And despite the exterminator's having kept his second appointment, he had not solved our flea issues.

With Wednesday, new worries arrived. The tremor in Ben's hands had worsened to the point where he had no control of his grip. His nurse reported that he'd slept okay through the night but couldn't hold his utensils at breakfast, so she'd had to feed him.

The team of doctors looped me into an early morning conference call. While the Swan-Ganz heart pump was ensuring stable numbers, his kidney function was deteriorating slightly, so they were calling in a nephrologist, inserting a Foley catheter, and debating whether dialysis would improve things.

I found the tremor the most demoralizing because it meant he couldn't hold his phone, and he certainly didn't have the fine motor skills necessary to dial. Nor could he manage his hearing aids. How would we be able to talk with each other? *Would* we be able to talk with each other?

In an effort to clear my head, I took a walk along the water's edge to watch the birds and look for dolphins and ran into a neighbor walking her Boykin spaniel. She kindly asked how things were going. After I laid a lot of the morning's report at her feet, she suggested that even though it all seemed overwhelming, the kidney issue appeared to be a manageable episode. "And it sounds like he's got a good team figuring out how to resolve it." Just having shared my fears made it possible for me to breathe more easily for the rest of the morning.

By midafternoon, however, the issues were of a different order of magnitude. A neurologist called to explain that there were growing concerns not only about those tremors but also about Ben's altered mental state and some behavioral changes. As the doctor explained, all this could be related to his kidney numbers going up. They were going to put an electroencephalograph on him and possibly do an MRI.

"Wait a minute! Ben can't undergo a standard MRI—he has a pace-maker. He's had issues with MRIs having to be aborted because his bad circulation made it impossible to track his pulse properly. Does his chart show the one he got a couple of months ago, even though it was done at a different hospital? Or you can look through the medical files he brought with him when he was admitted—they should be right there in his hospital room."

But were they? He'd already moved at least three times that I knew of, and not having visited him, I had no idea whether all the stuff Ben had Lamar load into the Suburban twelve days earlier had moved with him.

I refused to give up trying to reach him on his phone. First it was off completely, so no texts or messages were getting through. And then when he turned it on, he was too groggy to stay awake, so he'd say "Hello," sort of, and then he'd drop the phone and fall back asleep. The nurse stepped in midday to prompt him to stay awake and listen to my questions (and the answers often required her prompting as well). It was like talking with someone who's really drunk, asking him repeatedly to concentrate and stay in the moment. When the nutritionist came in to talk about his appetite in general, he thought she wanted to talk about lunch or dinner. I ended up hanging up so that perhaps with one less distraction he'd be better able to comprehend her role and provide her with the information she needed.

Somehow, he did manage to call me on his own at the end of the afternoon, but on a scale of 1 to 10, his ability to communicate was an unnerving 1.0. From that point forward, we would be dependent upon the nursing staff to facilitate any phone calls or FaceTimes.

It was becoming clear that I needed the people who loved him but weren't receiving the blow-by-blow reports to understand the severity of Ben's situation.

Our sons were being amazingly supportive from afar, networking with each other and tag-teaming their calls with me, aware of all the ups and downs, better at hearing what I couldn't verbalize, and leading with questions regarding how I was holding up.

But beyond this inner circle, I was besieged with calls and texts and emails focused solely on cheerleading, telling me, "Oh, Ben's tough; he's gonna be fine; he's doing great." Because they were so far removed from Ben's and my daily reality, the communications were rubbing me raw, and many of those same folks were emailing and phoning Ben directly, leaving messages that he was no longer capable of retrieving. I could tell from his desktop computer that he hadn't checked email in several days and was certain that meant he wasn't checking texts, either.

I agonized over how best to share what was going on. I didn't want to burden or alarm anyone, but at the same time, the situation had grown critical, and false optimism wasn't in anyone's best interests, especially not Ben's and mine.

The day had gone so poorly that I didn't get to meditation until late. Its focus was how to grow in trust and belief, recognizing one's true self as inspired and wise, and included some wisdom from Buddhist teacher Chögyam Trungpa: "Real fearlessness is the product of tenderness. It comes from letting the world tickle your heart, your raw and beautiful heart. You are willing to open up, without resistance or shyness, and face the world. You are willing to share your heart with others."

I thought of Ben's raw and beautiful broken heart and begged all his angels in that cone of light to help him hang on.

Wednesday, April 8
Ben update

Hi, all—

Ben has been undergoing some challenges since getting the balloon pump on Monday. The procedure itself went smoothly, but his kidney function is out of whack, which is manifesting itself in a variety of symptoms, including overwhelming grogginess and general confusion.

He has not looked at emails or phone messages since Monday morning. He had a brief window of looking at texts yesterday afternoon, but he found them confusing. There are some tremors in his hands that make it hard to put in his hearing aids, hold his phone, or type.

So his team has expanded to include neurologists and nephrologists who are working to get him back on an even keel over the course of the next 24 to 48 hours.

As one friend says, as upsetting and frustrating as this feels, it is a manageable episode. The doctors are confident it can be successfully resolved, and the neurologist assured me that everyone on the team is looking out for him.

xoxoxo SAC

***

No surprise—when I woke up Thursday, I was unable to get back to sleep. I'd learned that if I called the nurses' station before 5:30 a.m., whoever had worked the night shift usually had time to bring me up to date on how Ben was doing. But if it was later than that, I'd do best to wait until eight thirty or nine, after the shift change and doctors' rounds. During those intervening hours, I'd sit on the porch and stare at the stars.

That Thursday morning, even though sunrise wasn't until after 7:00 a.m., I was too late to make the predawn call. At loose ends, I took the time for the day's meditation. The focus was finding "a reason to hope in every situation," and the introduction included the observation that "the more grateful you are, the more hopeful you are." It also suggested that gratitude expands awareness; therefore, you should celebrate and praise whatever shows up in your life.

It was a struggle, but by dinnertime I was determined to celebrate and praise that day's phone call with Ben. He was doing marginally better, still confused when we talked but at least capable of some back-and-forth, and all before the day's dialysis, which the doctors expected would make a significant positive difference. I needed to recognize and accept that this long-distance process of supporting him through whatever came was going to be a roller coaster of good days and bad days. This had been one of the better ones, thanks be to God.

Make that a roller coaster of good hours and bad hours . . .

Late that night, a doctor called to let me know that because of Ben's ongoing compromised kidney function, the team wanted to start him on "slow" dialysis via a catheter in his thigh.

"Are you calling me for consent?"

"Yes, and I have a nurse here with me as a witness."

"My name is Sarah Cart. I am the wife of Benjamin Cart. His birthdate is . . . I understand you want to insert a catheter in his thigh in order to put him on slow dialysis. You have my consent."

James Reflects

When Dad told me he had congestive heart failure, I didn't really know how to feel. He seemed sad and obligated to let me know about it, but he made it sound like it was something the doctors were just keeping an eye on. I should have considered the source, Dad being as optimistic as he is, but it was definitely a blow.

That probably made it harder when I found out, in the spring of 2020, that Dad was in the hospital and wasn't coming out alive unless it was with a new heart. Was my last memory of him going to be his scootering into Disney after the fireworks show, cussing under his breath at all the people leaving, blocking the streets, while we were headed in for one last hurrah? I guess it could have been worse, but the act of considering what my last memory of him would be made me profoundly uneasy.

CHAPTER 6

Bearing the Weight
of Good Friday

April 10, 2020—April 15, 2020

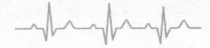

I needed to expand the phrase "good days and bad days" to include "long days."

Friday was one of those. Again, I woke up early and couldn't get back to sleep, but this time I was early enough to call Ben's nurse for a 5:00 a.m. update. She told me there was talk of putting in a second heart pump to augment Thursday night's slow dialysis.

Knowing Jon would be on a physician's schedule and thus well into his workday, I texted him despite the early hour. He called back so I could ask him a slew of questions before consenting to a second pump if and when the cardiology team called.

> ### April 10 (Good Friday), 11:00 a.m.
> ### Another stopgap procedure
>
> Hi, all—
>
> Because Ben's kidney function remains significantly compromised and
> he has other continuing issues with his overall well-being, today the
> doctors plan to insert an additional, stronger pump in Ben's heart.
>
> Whether they plan to replace the balloon pump from Monday or have
> the two pumps work together depends on how this morning's echocar-
> diogram is interpreted. Jon and I talked very early this morning, and he
> provided good questions to ask when the doctors call me for consent.
>
> I was able to speak with Ben briefly around 9:00 a.m. Although he is
> tired and remains confused, his mood is generally good. He is experi-
> encing some discomfort, but that seems to be directly related to all the
> various tubes, catheters, and monitors he's attached to.
>
> xoxoxo SAC

When the consent request came just before noon, however, it was
from a radiology tech, not a cardiologist. She had a nurse with her as a
witness. Would I give consent for a kidney biopsy so the doctors could
figure out whether Ben's kidneys were failing because of his autoimmune
disease or his congested heart?

"But I thought there was talk of a second pump."

"That may be, but the doctors would like to do this first."

"And then the pump later today?"

"You'll have to ask them; I can have someone give you a call if you'd
like."

"Yes, please. Oh, and you called for consent."

I was getting good at this.

"I am Benjamin Cart's wife, Sarah Cart. His birthdate is . . . I
understand that you want to do a kidney biopsy to determine whether
his kidneys are failing as a result of congestive heart failure or as a result
of his systemic sclerosis. I give my consent for this procedure."

Because I'd been having issues with my cell phone (it and the new house did not seem to get along), I asked the radiology tech to be sure the doctors called the landline. But that meant I needed to stay home and wait for the call. The minutes ticked by slowly. I sat down at the coffee table in the living room, cordless phone at my side, to work on a small, intricate wooden jigsaw puzzle that a lifelong Poconos friend had sent a couple of weeks earlier.

Finally, around two thirty, the call came. I picked up on the first ring. "Hi, Sarah. It's Debbie, Ben's transplant coordinator."

The tenor of her voice terrified me.

"Debbie—hi. I was expecting to hear from one of the doctors. Is Ben okay?"

"He is, but you need to know that because of his kidney issues, an internal hold has been placed on his status."

"Does that mean you're taking him off the list?"

"Not quite, but yes, for now—basically, yes. The doctors feel that transplantation would be unwise at this time."

"But when the biopsy results come back, depending on what they find, he can go right back on?"

"The team will have to discuss his case and agree to that."

"Similar to the process when they put him on the list in the first place? One of those once- or twice-a-week meetings?"

"Yes, similar to that."

"So this internal hold will be in place for a while?"

"Probably, yes."

Although the jigsaw puzzle had been coming together nicely, I didn't seem able to get any more pieces to fall into place, and despite having sent out an email that morning, I was going to have to craft a follow-up message—one that had to be sent before anyone called with holiday weekend greetings, if possible, because this was news that would be easier for me to write than to verbalize.

As I stared at my computer, the phone rang again. It was one of the cardiologists wanting to be sure I fully understood the purpose of the biopsy and the implications of the results.

"Do you have the results back already?"

"No. They're just starting the procedure now. The results should come in tonight."

"Is there any chance that based on what they show, you'll put him back on the list right away?"

"It's more about figuring out exactly what Ben needs and determining his best options. We're hoping the biopsy shows whether his kidneys are failing because his heart is failing or because of his autoimmune issues. Depending on that, we'll determine whether it's better for him to get a heart transplant or get a heart *and* a kidney transplant."

I went numb. "How does that work?"

"It's more common than you think. One donor. Two organs."

"Is the wait longer?"

"Not necessarily. It's just a question of when a match that works for Ben is found."

"But if a match were found this weekend?"

"He's not eligible at the moment. We need his kidney numbers to improve."

"And the second heart pump?"

"Probably tomorrow. The Swan-Ganz balloon will remain, and we'll put in a right-side Impella pump."

"And then he'll get back on the list?"

"When the team feels he's strong enough, the internal hold will be removed."

April 10, 4:00 p.m.
Glitches for Ben

Hi, all—

Ben's status on the transplant list is now on hold.

The situation evolved a few times.

It began with a predawn notice that he was going to get an additional heart pump. An echo was performed.

Then the doctors called for a kidney biopsy as well; that needed to wait until some medications were out of his system, and thus the biopsy couldn't happen until after 2:00 p.m. (fortunately, a relatively easy procedure).

As he went in for that, the doctor called to explain they are trying to determine if his kidney issues are related to congestive heart failure or if Ben's systemic sclerosis found a new place to settle in. They expect the results sometime late tonight.

They will likely put a pump in the right side of his heart tomorrow.

If it turns out that the kidney issues are related to systemic sclerosis, the path forward would be a joint heart and kidney transplant. If the issues are "just" congestive heart failure, then a new heart should be enough.

But before his status on any transplant list can be reactivated, his kidney function has to improve.

So last Friday we started a waiting game; a week in, the rules have changed a bit.

Despite its being a holiday weekend, I'm hoping that a solid few days of symptom management will warrant removing the hold from his status when the team convenes to reevaluate next week.

xoxoxo SAC

I went to our bedroom and started reading through the transplant book again with a whole new perspective. This kind of situation was in there. I'd read all those sentences before, but now they weren't merely describing a scenario; they were describing Ben's immediate reality.

A nurse helped Ben call me after the biopsy. He was beside himself. He wanted me to explain what was going on. He kept obsessing over having been "removed" from the list. It took a long time to get him calm enough to listen.

"It's temporary. Right now, your kidneys need to start responding to the dialysis."

"But first I need a pump and then I need a kidney transplant, and then I'll have to recover from that before they'll let me get a heart."

"No. That's not how it works. You'll probably get that other pump tomorrow. *If* they determine that you need a kidney transplant, when you get the kidney, you'll get a heart at the same time. But we don't know that you need one. Let's just see what the biopsy shows and how you feel once they get the pump in and the dialysis gets some of the water out of your system."

"I'm not happy." Spoken like a distraught ten-year-old boy.

"I know. I'm sorry. I love you."

The sky was dark when I hung up. In all the years I'd known him, I had never heard Ben so down.

I'd started the day with a call to Jon and ended the day with another. Presuming that I had already googled "Impella" (I had), he explained that this would be an "off-label use" of the pump—semantically alarming, but not unheard of or even unusual. While the literature talks about the device's efficiency in terms of hours, the clinic would be planning for the pump to serve as a bridge for however long it took to find a donor.

"But how likely is that, what with COVID and his being O negative, which means he's in line with every single other person on the list?"

"Sarah: because of COVID, the only people getting transplants at this point are those who are already hospitalized, because doctors can't be sure that people who are waiting at home are COVID-free, and no one has the capability to test them quickly. Ben is in the best place he can be right now. By the way, how high is his creatinine?"

"I don't know. Why?"

"Is he still making urine?"

"I don't think so."

"Even if he doesn't end up needing a double-organ transplant, until his kidneys are working well again, the doctors will have to hold off on prescribing Prograf—the heart-specific immunosuppressant—post-transplant."

I hung up, disconcerted by the fact that Easter weekend had arrived, but because of the coronavirus, there would be no Stations of the Cross, no Great Vigil, no sunrise service, no egg hunts, no bonnets or feasts or chocolate bunnies.

No family.

No Ben.

But under the circumstances, he was in the best place he could be.

The kidney biopsy results came Saturday morning and brought (relatively) good news: the damage was attributable to congestive heart failure, not systemic sclerosis, and his numbers were *slowly* improving, so there didn't appear to be a need for a kidney transplant. And that meant they could proceed with the insertion of the Impella pump on Ben's right side.

Six hours later, word arrived that the new device was in and all had gone well.

Saturday, April 11
Ben update

Hi, all—

Ben and I only got to exchange hellos as he was heading into today's pump-insertion procedure, and so he was already a bit sedated, but there is some encouraging news:

All went smoothly in the cath lab, and the second pump is in.

Also, the kidney biopsy showed that the issues are heart-related, not systemic sclerosis, and his numbers are getting better. While he will continue to receive dialysis 24-7 for now, at this time, HE DOES NOT NEED A KIDNEY TRANSPLANT.

So now we let the blessed folks in the surgical ICU give him the TLC he needs through this holiday weekend and wait to see what the new week brings when it gets here.

In the meantime, I've been looking forward for days to hearing Andrea Bocelli perform in the Duomo di Milano (he considers it a prayer and asks all to join him at 1:00 p.m. Eastern, streaming live on YouTube) and am sending each of you love and best wishes for an Easter full of blessings.

xoxoxo SAC

I waited until noon on Easter Sunday to call the hospital for an update. Ben's day nurse reported that his BUN (blood urea nitrogen) was down to 33 from 40 (goal: around 20), and his creatinine was down to 2.24 from Saturday's 2.59 (goal: around 1.2). She also noted that his answers to basic questions ("Do you know where you are?" "Do you know what year it is?") were correct, except that he kept insisting it was December. She helped him talk with me briefly; his ability to communicate had improved slightly to maybe 1.5, but he was complaining that his phone needed to be charged and he didn't know where the cord was.

Although I had taken several calls from family and friends, I struggled, unable to say "Happy Easter." I was grateful for the Bocelli concert and, once again, the three-week meditation experience. This day's focus was "the reality of inner strength" and provided nourishment for my soul, vital reminders for dealing with the ongoing anxiety over the unreal reality that I could not be with Ben as he was drifting away.

"True strength is rooted in inner peace and a sense of security."

"Breathe to find calm in the midst of chaos."

"Being at peace is my greatest strength."

"Expansive consciousness dissolves obstacles . . . Walk through it."

"Your greatest struggle will produce your greatest strength . . . In openness, there is strength."

At 4:00 p.m., my cell phone rang, and the screen read NO CALLER ID, but I answered it anyway. It was a different transplant coordinator, someone I hadn't spoken with before. Maybe she said her name was Sophia?

In the briefest of conversations, but one of the best, she stated simply, "He's back on the list."

Thanks be to God.

> **April 12**
> **Easter update re: Ben**
>
> Hi, all—
>
> Don't mean to drag all of you through every low and high of this roller-coaster ride, so today's report will be brief.
>
> Although Ben is still fairly out of it and finds communicating a challenge, the doctors reported this morning that his numbers are improving.
>
> And thanks to the steady dedication of all the folks looking after him in the surgical ICU, I received an unexpected Easter phone call a little bit ago:
>
> HE IS BACK ON THE LIST.
>
> So it has turned out to be a happy Easter. Thanks be to God.
>
> xoxoxo SAC

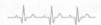

Some nights I would wake to the clock chiming a couple of rooms away, which meant either I'd slept past the early morning hours or it hadn't even gotten to be 11:00 p.m. or midnight yet. My sleep patterns had evolved: now I was waking for my first-light musings and panics and, if possible, that early call before the changeover from the night to day shift, when the team would have more time to provide information if they had it.

The Monday morning report was that Easter night they had to give him the narcotic Dilaudid because he'd gotten agitated when they went to change the dressings on his ankles. His kidney numbers were still down (BUN 25; creatinine 1.92), even as they'd slowed the dialysis flow, which meant his kidneys were stepping back up to do their job. A new possible glitch was that his hemoglobin had fallen from 8.9 to 7.6. His blood pressure, always low since the August 2018 diagnosis of congestive heart failure, was 109/65.

As I hung up from talking with the nurse, I was struck by how wonderfully generous so many people were being in their praise of my "strength" as this situation continued to evolve.

But as I sat at my desk imagining what it would have been like had Ben *not* ended up in the hospital and we were dealing with all the COVID isolation parameters and continuing to try to manage his wound care, sleep issues, and confusion—*that* would have been terrifying and an unbelievable disaster. Those last ten days when he was home, unable to stay awake long enough to date a document he'd just signed; falling off the commode and hitting his head; talking nonsense at 4:30 a.m. as he ate an unpeeled banana as if it were a T-bone and alternating bites of that with tomato and peanut butter—*that* had been *hell*.

This was not easy by any means. It was an exercise in heartbreak and frustration, especially with his present inability to communicate because of pain and pain management as well as compromised kidney function. But I knew at my core that Ben was in the best place he could be—a place where all those issues could be identified and addressed.

I patted myself on the back, said a prayer for Ben, and expressed gratitude to the universe.

Way to go, me.

Hang in for the long haul, Ben.

And blessings to all the folks who were helping us along the way.

I didn't expect my morning epiphany would be tested so soon.

By that evening, Ben's ability to interact with me had diminished to 0.5. Among a cluster of around nine attempted phone calls to his cell phone, the only one that got answered was the first, and he hung up approximately three seconds in. When I got through to his nurse, she explained, "There's this thing called ICU delirium." I broke down, weeping over the fact that we hadn't been together in seventeen days or had a real conversation in more than ten—I must have sounded like quite the hothouse flower, but she was patient as she let me rant myself out.

After hanging up, I compounded the pain by looking the ailment up on the internet. The best treatment? Visits with family, a loving touch, a whispered word in the ear.

But . . . COVID.

So we were left with FaceTime, dependent upon the nurses to facilitate. Graciously, that same nurse made a point of charging Ben's iPad, then Tuesday morning's nurse proved resourceful at setting aside a moment for us to speak for around five minutes right after breakfast.

Ben had a scruffy beard, all sorts of leads on his head, and tubes and wires in his neck and arms, but it was *wonderful* to see him, even as he kept closing his eyes and saying, "Talk to me. Tell me what you know." I resolved that for the next session I'd have a script, because any mention of the need for him to stay strong and upbeat until the arrival of a new heart was met quickly with "So they have a new heart?!?"

I was going to need stories about our boys and the grands, about Savvy, the birds, the lakes, fish, the full moon. Maybe read him some of the notes I'd emailed his way weeks earlier that had probably remained unread. Anything to keep up his spirits and anchor him to reality.

I went out for a walk to clear my head, bought a get-well card, stuffed it with family photos, and mailed it overnight so he'd get it ASAP and so the nurses could engage him in conversation about all of us.

As I walked home, I realized that any day he was on "the list" was a good day, worthy of gratitude.

By the afternoon shift, our next FaceTime (although it was on a hospital iPad because Ben's had been put away for safekeeping) proved a bit more successful because I was better prepared: I read him messages from folks from all areas of our lives and shared a photo of a rat snake eating an iguana, asking if he could tell what it was. His nurses had to coach him on the answers to some of my other questions, but not that one. And bless them for having shaved him, so he wore only a five o'clock shadow.

I lulled myself to sleep that night repeating, "All is well. All will be well."

At 9:00 a.m. on Wednesday, one of Ben's doctors called to provide "a general update." It was a brutally sobering conversation. I had already gone online and looked at Ben's numbers on his medical chart, noting that they weren't quite as good, but they didn't strike me as worrisome. I was wrong.

The doctor summarized the latest entries: Ben's weakening heart was being supported now with left and right heart pumps. His right-side pressures remained elevated, which meant they were continuing to remove fluid via dialysis. His central venous pressure was not improving and remained elevated, in the low 20s when it should be between 10 and 12 (whatever that meant).

His "mentation" had become a significant issue. Although he seemed a bit more awake, he answered questions very slowly. This may have been related to his kidney function, or it may have been a result of reduced blood flow to the brain. His kidneys had not improved as much as the doctors would have liked.

His lungs were okay, and he was "tolerating" food. His liver function was okay. His toes were purplish, so the circulation to his extremities was obviously compromised. They were going to continue his IV antibiotics for the time being.

But ominously, the doctor concluded by emphasizing that Ben's mental capacity and kidneys needed to improve. Now.

"It is a tenuous and dynamic situation."

I hung up the phone knowing that the doctor had left a lot unsaid. He was preparing me to learn in the next day or two that Ben was no longer a candidate for transplant, and I wondered how in the world I was going to manage to get the powers that be (who were they?) to let me see him in spite of COVID, however briefly, to thank him for all he had taught me about love, endurance, and greeting every situation with openness and faith. To tell him I so admired the fight he had put up. To let him hear me whisper "I love you" in his ear one last time, and to say goodbye.

A couple of hours later, Nurse Michelle facilitated a brief FaceTime session for us that proved excruciatingly challenging—Ben could hardly stay awake or focus. Since it wasn't going well, she suggested we try again later, sometime when he was more alert. My heart ached as I left the timing up to her to orchestrate.

Finally, around 2:15 p.m., she was able to connect us for another FaceTime. Then she turned the camera so I was looking at her masked face.

"The transplant coordinator, Jessica, just walked into the room; would it be okay to bring her into this conversation?"

I didn't want to panic, but after Good Friday's frightening call from Debbie and this morning's unsettling conversation with the doctor, the request unnerved me.

But the nurse's eyes were smiling. Was that sympathy? Concern? Support? She turned the lens toward Jessica, who was also masked. And smiling.

"I am so glad I have the two of you together," Jessica said. "There's news. A heart has been allocated."

"Excuse me?" A shiver ran through me; I wasn't sure I could breathe.

"We have a heart."

CHAPTER 7

"This Is 50 Percent of the Battle"

April 15, 2020—April 18, 2020

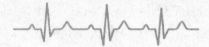

Jessica apologized for not being able to stay and talk. There were several items she needed to follow up on right then, but she promised she'd give me a quick call in half an hour or so, and she'd be back in the early evening to answer any questions Ben or I might have.

Nurse Michelle explained that she, too, had a checklist to put Ben through—everything from paperwork to blood tests—beginning right away, with no more fluids or ice. But she promised that Ben and I would be able to talk later.

As soon as we hung up, I texted Jon to ask how the timing of a transplant works once a heart has been found. Rather than typing out a response to my text, he called within moments, and thanks to his input, I understood that all this was going to take many hours, if not more than a day. Jon also helped me draw up a list of questions for Jessica when she and I spoke shortly thereafter:

"What are the chances that this is a dry run?"

"How many transplant centers with patients higher on the list are you waiting to hear from?"

"Where is Ben on the clinic's list?"

Calmly and clearly, Jessica explained that Dr. Cedric Sheffield, the surgical director of the heart transplant program at the clinic, was preparing to collect the heart that evening. She added, "There are a lot of variables that still need to fall into place before we can determine the timing. While it's possible he'll decide upon seeing it that the match won't work, that's a decision he will make quickly, practically as soon as he sees it. We will let you know that immediately. But right now, I can tell you this much: as of this moment, the heart is specifically allocated to Ben."

When Ben and I spoke again that evening, adrenaline made him more coherent than he'd been in a week, and we discussed when to share the news with others. He was keyed up and wanted to broadcast it near and far; I maintained that we should wait until confirmation came, because it wouldn't be fair to get everyone's hopes up in case this was a false start. I promised Ben that the moment he went into surgery I would convey the news to the boys, his mother, his sister, and the rest of the family along with our closest friends. Reluctantly, he agreed, then declared that he wanted me to stay on the phone with him until they came to take him to the OR. I finally convinced him that we should ask the nurse what, from her experience, she might be able to predict about the timing.

"It will be hours before a decision is made, and then the heart needs to be brought to the clinic. Best guess is that surgery won't begin until late morning. Right now, Ben, you need to sign this bit of paperwork, then it would be good if you could try to get some sleep."

That meant she considered him coherent enough to provide his own consent. My heart swelled. We said good night, knowing full well we'd likely talk again soon.

Of course Ben couldn't go to sleep right away; he was far too excited. Then one of the transplant surgeons stopped in to see him, and afterward, Ben explained to the nurse that he needed to call me again and send an email.

The phone conversation was brief: "Dr. Sheffield came by to tell me he's flying out tonight and coming back in the morning!"

The email was briefer. Addressed to me, his mother, and his sister, it consisted of the misspelled subject line "Cedric is afligt." No message.

Dammit, Ben—we agreed we weren't going to tell anyone in case this heart isn't the right one for you! I thought.

Ben's mother immediately "replied all," commenting on his typo and the fact that the body of the email was blank, and shortly thereafter, his sister wondered, "Isn't there a Cedric in *Harry Potter*?"

I held off on responding, hoping they'd think that perhaps since it was late I was already in bed. But I couldn't get to sleep, either. Around 11:00 p.m., Jessica texted an update: as things stood, they expected a final go or no-go decision from the surgeon around 6:00 a.m., at which point they planned to take Ben into the operating room for pre-op procedures.

Knowing the next day would be a long one, I made myself stay in bed. Breathing in and out slowly, repeating "A miracle; a heart," finally enabled me to doze a bit, but at 5:00 a.m. I gave in to the urge to call the nurses' station for an update. They put me through to Jessica (when would she be allowed to sleep?), who reported that the collection was due to happen in the next hour or so. "There are several organs and several recipients, so they have to wait until all the surgeons are there before they can begin," she said. She also told me that Ben would be taken into the operating room shortly, even though the surgery itself likely wouldn't begin until 9:00 a.m.

An hour and a half later, the landline rang. It was Jessica.

"This is not a dry run. The heart is due on-site at 10:00 a.m. You can expect that Ben will be in surgery until around 3:00 p.m."

Ten minutes later, Dr. Nicolas Brozzi, the surgeon who would implant the heart, called to touch base. "Ben is in the operating room being prepped. The whole team is ready, and things are looking good.

This is a wonderful and exciting step, but know that this is only fifty percent of the battle. Recovery will be the other fifty percent.

"Try not to worry; I will call you when the surgery is complete."

James Reflects

Right before Dad went in for surgery—we had just gotten the call—I remember not knowing what to say but feeling like it was the last time I was going to be able to say something to him. We're not a family that says the word "love" a lot, and I just really needed to tell him that I love him before he went in.

I hit Send on a text and didn't know if he got it or if I would get a reply—ever. But he did respond with a great big "I love you too," and I just broke down and bawled. I don't remember where I was, but I do remember being unable to stop crying for a while and feeling overwhelmed.

Thursday, April 16, 7:00 a.m.
GOOD MORNING! THERE IS A HEART!

Hi, all—

A long day ahead.

The heart has passed all tests with the surgeon, so this is real (not a dry run, which happens 10–20% of the time).

Ben is headed into the OR now to be prepped. Hopefully there will be news late this afternoon.

Cart family tradition through the generations when wishing good luck has always been to say, "We are pointing the dog eye at you!" meaning a dowsing stick. So please, all: point the dog eye toward Ben today and through the recovery to come.

xoxoxo SAC

The day's meditation was about "living by the light of hope." It could not have felt more timely or right. In the introduction, Deepak Chopra explained that the energy of hope opens you to calmness, clarity, and power, and he cautioned against dimming hope for others. The centering mantra was "My future unfolds with hope and joy."

I paid bills and answered the dozens of emails, texts, and phone calls that arrived in response to my 7:00 a.m. email blast, then took a long walk to get a few errands done, and finally arrived home to wait. And wait. And take more phone calls.

Savvy knew something was up: she Velcroed herself to my side, giving one or two solid thumps of her tail whenever our eyes met. I was glad she'd been flea-free for weeks and that it finally seemed like the house and I were too.

At three fifteen, Dr. Brozzi called.

"Surgery went well. It is a good heart and a good fit. He will be on the ventilator for a couple of days, and the balloon remains in for now to help the new heart adjust. Dialysis also continues."

"What's become of his pacemaker?"

"It's gone. He doesn't need it anymore."

It was day 34 of the pandemic, the first day of Ben's new life.

April 16, 3:20 p.m.
GOOD AFTERNOON!

Hi, all—

The doctor just called to report that Ben is out of surgery, and it went well.

"A beautiful heart, a good heart, a good fit," but the next three to four days will be critical.

He will be on a ventilator for a couple days, and they expect he will be fairly out of it for that period. The pump that was inserted just last Saturday has been removed and is gone; the balloon pump that went in early last week will remain for now to help as the new heart adjusts.

The slow dialysis will continue for a while; his old pacemaker (installed September 2018) is now a thing of the past.

Time to pray for his swift recovery and say a prayer, too, for a devastated family's having given us a wonderful gift.

xoxoxo SAC

By late afternoon, I'd received scores of texts and emails full of prayers: of gratitude, for a speedy recovery, and for a suffering family who had graciously and generously turned their loss into our miracle. Keeping in mind the surgeon's caution that the surgery was only half the battle and that recovery would be the other half, I could only feel relief that this new battle was underway at last. And as a lifelong friend of Ben's pointed out in a congratulatory text, with a new heart, Ben could fall in love with me, and me with him, all over again.

As evening fell, Ben's nurse reported that he was alert when he came back from the operating room and included the news that, based on her experience with other patients, if the ventilator tube came out the next day, maybe they'd get him up and walking, even as she reminded me of the critical nature of the ensuing ninety-six hours. Giving thanks for miracles but exhausted, I went to bed early and got the best night's sleep I'd had in nearly a year.

Friday morning's meditation focused on "the inner child reborn," and I marveled at what felt like appropriate timing—this was like a rebirth for Ben.

But how quickly I had forgotten that we were still on the battlefield; instead of marveling at this new beginning, I should have been bracing myself.

I waited hopefully for word that the ventilator had been removed and Ben was out of bed, but the nurses had their hands full with his immediate needs and could only enable two twenty-second FaceTimes over the course of the day. As uplifting messages of joy and support and prayers poured in from friends and family, many calling it the best news they'd heard since the chaos of the pandemic took over everyone's lives, I was beginning to realize, now that he was in the surgical ICU, tracking down complete and timely updates on his condition had grown exponentially more challenging.

In the ten days since he'd last been able to use his phone unassisted, I'd fallen into a pattern of calling the nurses' station three times a day: early morning, midday, and late afternoon. And fairly regularly, doctors or techs had reached out to obtain consent. Now, however, even though it was only day 1 of Ben's recovery, there had been a marked shift. I was getting put on hold, listening to earworm music for ten minutes, and getting disconnected. If no one answered after eight rings, I'd hang up, my stomach clenching, pulse racing, and imagination heading down dark alleys. When they did answer, though, I'd be forwarded to whoever was Ben's nurse at that time, hoping he or she would pick up before I got disconnected again. With each failure, I tried to swallow the frustration or breathe through it, then resolve to try again later and look for a distraction.

There had been one nurse a week earlier who'd said that legally she couldn't answer some of my questions and advised me to access Ben's online patient portal to check his test results, which I'd found unnerving. Was I really expected to interpret those results on my own? But with so many other personnel reaching out and providing answers as various procedures needed my approval, I hadn't dwelled on it. Now, needing to find a balance wherein I could feel informed and in touch without being a pest or a burden to the team consumed with caring for him, I was realizing it would be best if I always started there.

Oh, how I just wanted to *see* him and have him hear my voice.

The reason for the communication hassles was simple but not obvious: COVID, in addition to preventing patients from having visitors, prevented volunteers from reporting for duty. The surgical ICU nurses found themselves having to perform dozens of tasks not normally included in their staggering job descriptions: everything from delivering mail, answering phones, and taking messages to running errands and providing the often-overlooked niceties that enable patients and medical professionals to move through their days with grace.

What details might have been gleaned had it been possible to indulge in the luxury of sitting quietly at Ben's bedside?

With no word about the ventilator or getting Ben out of bed, my unease grew. Then I found a voice mail from the social workers who were going to oversee Ben's discharge from the hospital. The call hadn't rung through to my cell because of the hurricane-proof architecture of the new home. *That'll need to change*, I thought. The message explained that, rather than being "discharged to home," Ben would probably go into an intense two-week rehab program that specialized in educating transplant recipients.

When I returned the call, the social workers reiterated what we'd been told numerous times during the months we'd been working on getting Ben on "the list": because of the immunosuppressants, he would come home with little if any immune system. The COVID pandemic demanded a new layer of caution, and we would have to be hypervigilant. For at least six months, Ben would have to wear a mask, preferably an N95, anytime he left the house. There could be no houseguests or company. Any contractor or repairman entering our home would have to wear a mask as well. If I were to go out and about and run a bunch of errands, it would be best if I planned to change my clothes upon returning home.

And, they advised, since masks and latex gloves were now routinely out of stock, I should place orders immediately in the hope they'd be delivered before Ben arrived home. Although they couched their projection with "Every case is different," they expected he'd be headed to rehab "soon." Where was the rehab facility? In Hollywood, just south of Fort Lauderdale.

I wondered if there would be an opportunity at some point for hands-on instruction regarding caring for a transplant recipient. So much was up in the air because of COVID restrictions that they weren't sure. While I was glad to have a vague outline of what lay ahead for Ben, my unease increased.

It lessened slightly when a late afternoon call came through from the surgeon. He reported that Ben was coming along well, but the team needed to proceed slowly and carefully.

"He has a good strong heart." I felt relief at those words.

He went on to explain that based on the first twenty-four hours, the expectation was that Ben would have one more day of the balloon and the ventilator. When I asked about his kidneys, the word was that they were still shut down and that the situation could take weeks to resolve itself.

I hung up feeling slightly better, then found a mood-elevating email from business partner Mark: "Ben texted Wednesday night that he was okay and surviving the grind but that he must have missed the part about how hard the grind was going to be. Glad he is on to a 'new grind.' Thinking of you. All our best from snowy Ohio."

I, too, was glad Ben was on a "new grind."

**Friday, April 17
Full day no. 1**

Hi, all—

Ben had a good night last night and is doing just as the doctors had hoped. They are pleased. But they want to "take it slow," so he will be on the ventilator for another day or two (dozing most of that time), and dialysis will continue until his kidneys wake up.

Today's highlights came via FaceTime, thanks to his nurse.

This morning, she gave me a "tour" of his room—there is an AMAZING amount of equipment in there. It brought to mind 1960s movies about space travel with rooms full of IBM computers.

Then this afternoon he opened his eyes to say hello at my request. They were beautiful to see . . . thanks be to God.

xoxoxo SAC

The support I had been receiving from near and far astounded me: cards and letters, emails, phone calls, meals—I would never be able to convey the depth of my gratitude. Each gesture bolstered my strength, and I wanted to share that strength with Ben, hand it to him, envelop him in it, have it take root in his bones.

As Saturday dawned, Ben's night nurse told me that not only were his numbers relatively good but also that one of the medications, to help his lungs, had been cut back. He'd had to be sedated, however, because he was anxious—not unusual for a patient dealing with a breathing tube, yet still disconcerting to hear. I was desperate to see him, to touch his cheek, hold his hand, kiss his forehead (even if it had to be through a mask), but the COVID restrictions remained inflexible.

It struck me that maybe in a few more days Ben would be able to answer his phone by himself—oh, how wonderful that would be. But although no one had mentioned ICU delirium since Monday or said anything further about his mentation, I had no reason to think the surgery had resolved those issues. I was going to have to be patient.

In the meantime, I had hours to fill, and I tried to focus on gratitude for what was going right. As it happened, two lovely distractions landed in my email inbox from Jewels, a friend of Ben's sister, writing to share her hands-on experience, gleaned from having been a caregiver to her husband, Christopher, after his cardiac surgery.

In the first message, which carried the subject line "Once you get your heartthrob home," she recommended placing a baby monitor in his room. That gave me pause; it hadn't occurred to me that his room wouldn't be our room. But no matter: a monitor would be a good idea— that way, if he needed to nap, I wouldn't have to barge in to see how he was doing. As Jewels explained, "Christopher could communicate with me when he wanted to . . . moreover, he didn't need to take a painful big breath in order to call out." She went on to say that it was "a gentle way to communicate, and he really appreciated it."

She also said her husband found sitting up to be a painful challenge, and he experienced drenching sweats, so she kept a pile of clean fitted sheets on hand so the bed could be changed quickly. In addition, there were painful breathing exercises that had to be done daily, and just in case I'd never heard of it, post-op depression is relatively common for heart patients. In her case, she wrote, "it was helpful for me to be aware of the possibility as a caregiver and 'good wifey.'"

The second message carried the subject line "Some practical advice for handling meds and more."

This morning, I remembered the issue of handling all the meds once he got home. When the exhaustive list came in from the nurses, I put on my Spreadsheet Queen crown and converted everything ("take with food," "don't take with food"; "take every three hours," "take as needed," etc.) into a schedule. In addition to meds, I included mealtimes, breathing exercises, other exercises, and calls to various medical folks. It made life much easier.

As I built the spreadsheet, I left blank columns next to some meds in order to fill in the times those were actually taken. That whole process had to be fluid too, because he had some allergic reactions that meant we had to try other alternatives.

Also, some of the painkillers were highly regulated, which meant they required longer refill windows and were really slow to fill on weekends. And some of them and the antibiotics caused constipation, so it's important to keep a gentle softener like MiraLAX on hand.

I kept all his meds in a deep Tupperware bowl and glued paper circles over the caps, labeling each with the name and dosage so I could identify what was in each vial just by looking down from above instead of having to pull each one up and look at the pharmacists' labels on the sides. Eventually, as the number of pills diminished and I recognized which pill was which, I was able to transfer them into divided pill boxes for morning, noon, and night. He took that task over at around ten weeks.

Throughout, I kept repeating the mantra "What can Christopher do?" The goal was for him to feel more in control of his recovery process and less "taken care of," a fine line to walk. It was really important to talk with him about this as soon as his head started to become less fuzzy from the painkillers. A lot of sleep and daily exercise helped him recover pretty quickly.

Here endeth my brain drain.

Saturday, April 18
Full day no. 2

Hi, all—

Ben continues to do well, and his numbers continue to improve.

Today's big excitement was that they took out the remaining (balloon) pump, although for now the slow dialysis continues and he remains on the ventilator.

When the nurse facilitated FaceTime for me tonight, Ben's eyes were wide open. Because of the ventilator, however, he was not wearing his hearing aids, so it was really just an exchange of smiles. (But oh, wow, what a heartwarming exchange of smiles!)

Hope everyone is enjoying a wonderful weekend (it certainly feels wonderful at this end).

xoxoxo SAC

Saturday night, the order came to remove Ben's breathing tube, and once that task was accomplished, it was as if they'd let a genie out of a bottle. He was hyper and cajoled the night nurse into helping him send some texts and make a few FaceTime calls to our boys and me. Off the ventilator, he was hoarse, giddy, high on painkillers, disoriented, punch-drunk, a bit muddled, and so so so happy. While it was an amazing thrill to hear his voice, his confusion made me edgy, apprehensive about all I needed to learn regarding how best to care for him when he got home.

CHAPTER 8

The Slippery Slope

April 19, 2020—April 26, 2020

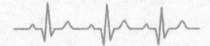

First thing Sunday, I got through to a terribly taciturn night nurse who wouldn't share any details about how Ben was doing, even after I explained I was his wife. She said she'd have the doctor call me. As the hours dragged on, I grew increasingly uneasy. When I'd heard nothing by noon, I called back, and the day nurse facilitated a brief FaceTime. That was only possible after Ben had explained to her how to hook his iPad into the hospital's Wi-Fi.

But despite having the wherewithal to resolve that situation, Ben was extremely confused. He didn't know who I was, although he appreciated that I knew everyone in his family.

"Please tell my mother and my sister that I'm okay."

Shaky, I asked his nurse to please have the doctor call me, then waited through the endless afternoon.

When the doctor was finally able to call, around 5:00 p.m., I begged him to tell me what was going on. After assuring me that "all is good with the new heart; it is strong and a good fit," his only counsel was "He will improve."

Yet less than twenty-four hours earlier, Ben had initiated communications with all of us and had been laughing, asking questions, and talking nonsensically about funny stuff. What had changed? Something was terribly wrong.

The nurse on duty at 5:30 a.m. Monday revealed that Ben didn't sleep at all during the night; perhaps someone would be able to give me more information after the doctors rounded.

When I called back at 11:20 a.m., the day nurse described him as "confused," with an elevated white blood count. Although Ben was sitting in a chair (oh, my goodness—he was finally out of bed!), he was on oxygen because there were "infiltrates" in his lungs, and the team had started him on an antibiotic. (A quick Google search after the call revealed that infiltrates could include any substance denser than air, such as blood, pus, or protein.) He was also on medication to support his blood pressure. His dialysis continued. The nurse mentioned they were doing some "troubleshooting." It appeared Ben was having aspiration issues and difficulty swallowing, and "sometimes he knows his name, but sometimes he doesn't." He would be going for a CT scan and a chest X-ray shortly and maybe getting outfitted with a feeding tube.

Panicked and in frustration, I reached out to Dr. Bush's office and begged his assistant for help: Ben's surgery had been four days previously, yet the majority of information I was getting was coming from the nursing staff—and only in response to my being a squeaky wheel, a role that made me highly uncomfortable. I'd heard from the social workers, who seemed to imply there was a timetable for his coming home, but the other bits and pieces I was hearing made it appear that a lot of things were slipping, quickly, in the wrong direction. What did "troubleshooting" mean? Why a CT scan? My head was about to explode.

As the one who was ultimately going to be responsible for caring for him once he got discharged, wasn't I part of the team? Why did it feel like I was in the locker room suited up for a home game and just learning that the squad left two days ago for an away match? Would it be possible, please, to have a doctor touch base with me on a daily basis to keep me up to date?

At 4:00 p.m. my landline rang. It was a Dr. Hernandez, who informed me he was going to be on Ben's rotation for the next two weeks and would be calling every day he was on duty to go over Ben's case (bless Dr. Bush's assistant). Finally, I was getting some answers, even as I found them alarming.

The CT scan had been to rule out a stroke. His white blood count was of concern. His kidneys were not kicking back in, but perhaps that would change by the end of the week. They'd had to start him on pro-phylaxis PCP—a regimen of drugs taken to help prevent pneumocys-tis pneumonia—"because of the infiltrates in his lungs. Can't have him coming down with that."

Monday, April 20
Full day no. 4

Hi, all—

Although much to his joy they took out his breathing tube on Satur-day, Ben remains terribly confused. As his nurse put it this afternoon, "Sometimes he knows his name, and sometimes he doesn't."

The dialysis in support of his kidneys continues. Not much has changed there recently, but the doctors hope that by the end of the week the situation will improve. He barely slept last night, however. And he is having some lung issues, so now he's on oxygen.

Plus, because he was coughing and choking and having trouble swal-lowing this afternoon, he also was evaluated by a speech pathologist and has ended up with a feeding tube. Jon has reassuringly pointed out that this is a benign and useful way to give him the calories he needs to heal.

Despite a collection of what feels like exhausting setbacks, all this is a massive improvement over what we were dealing with a week ago.

Perhaps it's time to reread *The Little Engine That Could.*

xoxoxo SAC

Tuesday proved the darkest day yet.

The nurse didn't pick up when I called at 5:45 a.m. I tried again thirty minutes later and learned Ben had finally had a good night's sleep, thanks to melatonin. They were getting lots of fluid off his kidneys every hour; he was on two antibiotics to help with breathing. But he was more confused: he didn't know where he was, and he had no idea of the year, much less the date.

A Dr. Torres called in the late morning, but as soon as I answered, he told me he couldn't stay on the line. Before hanging up, however, he assured me that Ben's heart was "doing fine." When he called back, he explained that Ben's lungs were not functioning well and that his arterial blood gases were at zero and not improving. They were going to have to escalate his treatment with a BiPAP ventilator. In addition, there were concerns regarding his mentation and airway. They wanted to reintubate.

"I have Dr. Ramirez here as a witness—"

"I am Benjamin Cart's wife, Sarah Cart. His birthdate is . . . I understand that you want to reintubate him to secure his airway. I give my consent for this procedure."

In his daily call, Dr. Hernandez reported that they'd gotten around 2.4 liters of fluid off his kidneys, thanks to dialysis, and another 1.4 liters via the chest tubes. "He has a young, healthy heart."

Early in the evening, Nurse Erica enabled a FaceTime session that left me devastated. Although Ben was heavily sedated and totally zonked, with his eyes rolled back into his head, she felt it would be good for me to see him and reported that his arterial blood gases were a little better.

By Wednesday, we'd reached day 6 of Ben's new heart. On day 4, he'd gotten a feeding tube; on day 5 they put him on a ventilator. I took a midmorning call during which I was told that the doctors wanted to order another chest X-ray and an immediate CT scan of his chest and abdomen to determine if there was an infection in his bloodstream—and they needed to change his dialysis catheter. The doctor who called to explain all that, Dr. Stefano, began by saying simply, "Something is not going right with him," then asked, "Do you give consent?"

"Yes! My name is Sarah Cart," and all the rest.

I was frustrated and confused—by the trending direction of Ben's "recovery," by the crushing flood of details, and by the feeling that if I could just spend some time in Ben's room with the members of the medical team, questions could be asked and answers given, and maybe, just maybe, I could get a grip on what was happening.

Too often it was taking me, Ben's wife and most passionate supporter, his supposed sole link to the outside world and future caregiver, more than half an hour to get through. And that evening, I learned of other people who had called the hospital and had been put through immediately to his nurses and had been made privy to details about which the hospital had yet to inform me.

What with the ventilator, intubation, catheters, and who knew what else, it felt like he was being tortured, while in our new home, out of the loop, unable to communicate with him, I was being tortured too. A week earlier, I'd been afraid we were going to lose him before a heart became available, but then we'd gotten our miracle. Now I was afraid we still might lose him. I was beside myself thinking that at the rate Ben was deteriorating, I (like too many families whose loved ones were dying of COVID) wouldn't be allowed to visit or say goodbye. The doctor assured me the time for that had not come.

"Something is not right, but all is great with the new heart."

Ben Reflects

There came a point when I finally just cratered and had to go on life support. But I was a little small physically, and that was part of the miracle for me. I'd shrunk down, whereas a lot of male heart transplant patients are big guys who need a physically big heart. That was less of a problem for me, so I had a lot more choices out there. All we ever heard from the doctors about the one I got was that it's "a young and healthy heart." We had no idea where it came from. They would not tell us.

Panicky, I called Jillian in Maine to vent and rant. For more than an hour, I absorbed all the TLC she could project my way.

I needed to count my blessings again. For friends far away, like Jillian, who dropped everything to take my calls and answer my texts when I was scared or falling apart. For local friends too, such as Mary and Geof, who regularly, lovingly, and generously included me in their fresh-air small-group gatherings, all four or five of us seated on folding chairs six feet from everybody else, dining off lap trays—they considered me part of their social COVID-free "bubble." For Cindy and Tim, a mile down the road, who thought of me in the midst of their dinner several evenings and each time set aside a plateful of food that was then delivered ready to eat the next day, complete with a couple dozen cookies on the side. For the several other great cooks—Angie, Didi, Terry, Suzanne, and Diane—who also continually kept me in their orbit. A batch of lentil soup. Spareribs. Baked ziti in Bolognese sauce. Enchiladas. For Sarina, who found creating masterpieces in her kitchen to be therapeutic during the ongoing lockdown. She'd call half an hour before dinnertime to schedule a drop-off of multicourse meals fresh from the oven or stovetop, ready to place on the table, or if that wasn't convenient, she packaged them to go into my freezer. For Honey, the cashier at our local market, whose loving smile warmed my heart (even though we'd never seen each other without masks) as she scanned the UPC codes on the bag of potato chips and screw-top bottle of Pinot Grigio on the occasional afternoon when the thought of heating a real meal or simply opening the fridge overwhelmed me.

Family and friends called and scheduled Zoom sessions and shared uplifting articles and videos. Many sent word of prayer circles and positive energy. I'd received scores of cards and letters and emails as well as care packages. Carrie had shipped an overflowing Easter basket from Hartford; a box of boutique chocolates had come from Hitomi in New York; and Jillian had sent chocolate chip blondies from Maine (labeled "for medicinal purposes; take as needed"). Plus, the hospital was receiving gifts and get-well messages for Ben too, even though the volunteers who usually distributed such items had been absent for weeks.

Then Ted, our third son, called, and he and I had a long midday phone conversation. He pointed out how amazingly blessed our whole family had been these past few months. Dad got his heart. No one had gotten COVID. He had wanted to quit his job in January to look for something new but *didn't* (now was not the time to be looking for work). He was happy to be in Boston while his younger brother, Benjamin, who *did* quit his job to take a new one just in time to avoid having to reschedule a major live musical event, remained safe in Nashville. His immediately older brother, William, was in a good spot out in the countryside rather than in his former seven-hundred-square-foot apartment in downtown Manhattan. His oldest brother, James, sister-in-law Ashley, and nieces and nephew were safe in western Massachusetts—perhaps going a little stir-crazy and disappointed by all the restrictions on their "normal" lives but making it work. And I did *not* have to have back surgery, nor was I holed up at our old house, but rather I was busy with productive projects settling into this new place, making it ready for when Ben returned home.

The world was shifting all around us and likely would never go back to the way it was, but we had been remarkably blessed. Remarkably, amazingly blessed.

Although I had been saying it often, at the very least I needed to say it again: thanks be to God.

William Reflects

My mom is great in a crisis; she might even thrive on it. I think she's one of those people who actually does better when the house is on fire a little bit. In fact, the more the house is on fire, the cooler and calmer she gets. When the house seemed like it was really going up, she kept chill and carried on in a way that I couldn't understand at the time. It was inspiring. She was not in denial. She displayed acceptance and perseverance in a way that I hope I can emulate in my own life.

Benjamin Reflects

My mother has always had a talent for keeping her cool in a crisis. She seems to really dial in and plan and coordinate what needs to happen. She made sure my dad got the best care possible, and that took a lot of persistence.

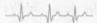

In the early afternoon I took a call from Dr. Hernandez. Ben still had the Swan-Ganz pump—the pulmonary-artery catheter. He wasn't producing urine. His blood pressure was low, so there was talk of increased medications, but they needed to hold off on giving him Prograf, the one immunosuppressant that would be critical for his transplanted heart for the rest of his life.

And then Dr. Stefano called with the results of the CT: the diffuse bilateral consolidation and infiltrates at the upper left and upper and middle right of Ben's lungs were worse than they were three days ago. (Had I heard this before? The details were suffocating me.) The team had also done ultrasounds of his lower legs and arms, all of which were "clean."

"Plus, um . . . one other thing." The doctor hesitated for a moment, then said, "The radiologist reading the CT scan wondered: Has anyone noticed that Ben, um, has a fractured left hip?"

"I'm sorry—what was that?"

"The radiologist set up the portable X-ray a little lower than usual and says Ben's left hip is fractured."

"Oh, wow." I paused as an image of Ben climbing out of Lamar's Suburban after one of his wound clinic visits, a cane in his hand, came into focus. "I might be able to explain that. He hurt it a few days before arriving at the hospital for this stay."

"How so?"

"He'd been having terrible sleep issues for months, and apparently he fell asleep on his way back to bed from the bathroom in the middle of the night and ended up on the floor."

"Apparently?"

"Well, I didn't know about it at the time. He'd taken to sleeping on the couch in the living room because he was so restless. He was afraid he'd fall out of bed, and the couch was closer to the floor—it's a long story, but yes, he fell and didn't say anything about it until I asked why he'd suddenly started taking so much ibuprofen. Then he admitted he'd fallen a couple of days earlier. I'd have to guess it was the weekend before he was admitted, so maybe March twenty-first or twenty-second."

"And he was getting around?"

"Yes, although he started using a cane, but I thought that was because of his infected ankles and that the fall just made it more obvious that a cane was a good thing."

"All right. We'll have to get orthopedics to evaluate him, but that can wait for now." Wednesday evening, I got another call, this one from a doctor who identified himself as "the other Dr. Hernandez." (Yes, there were two in the ICU—Dr. Luis Hernandez and Dr. Jaime Hernandez.) "I'm in charge of him for the coming week. He is extremely sick. He was severely compromised before the surgery. It will take some time for the damage done to his liver and kidneys by the congestive heart failure to resolve itself, and his lungs are struggling."

I was scribbling notes furiously, trying to keep up.

While Ben's blood pressure was improving, and his heart was moving in the right direction (meaning some medications could be reduced), his white blood count had jumped from the day before. The lung samples taken to assess infection had yet to yield any results. Ben was on antimicrobials, antifungals, and antivirals. There had been a dry cough when he was extubated; therefore he might remain intubated for another week or two, or the doctors might opt instead to perform a tracheostomy.

I was grateful for the doctor's candor, even as I was drowning in the particulars. And in the end, he threw me a life preserver. Ben's lungs were "better today than yesterday. This infection or inflammation or whatever it turns out to be is easily untangled with time and patience. You just need to understand that at the moment it's an all-hands-on-deck situation, and the SICU staff is here to address it."

Wednesday, April 22
Full day no. 6

Hi, all—

While Ben's new heart continues to behave just as the doctors had hoped it would, his recovery is hitting roadblocks on other fronts.

This week, each day has thrown in a new glitch. The extreme confusion and disorientation that led to Monday's feeding tube was followed yesterday by the need to reintubate him to protect his airway. Thus he is heavily sedated 100 percent of the time.

The issue prompting the introduction/reintroduction of those two devices has been aspiration, and unfortunately a CT scan today revealed that there is some stuff in his lungs. Even while they wait for culture results, they've started him on antibiotics in the hope of nipping whatever this is in the bud.

Also, in the midst of today's CT scan of his lungs and lower abdomen, they noticed a fracture in his left hip.

At least I was able to help solve that mystery: a middle-of-the-night fall about a week before he was admitted to the hospital. And while he occasionally mentioned pain at the time, he certainly didn't think he had broken anything. Because the pain abated once he was settled into the ICU (or at least was minimal compared to other issues he was having), he never mentioned it to the hospital staff.

The doctor indicated that the hip is not an immediate concern and may just result in some aches, pains, and stiffness once Ben is finally able to begin physical therapy.

Slow dialysis also continues as they wait for his kidneys to kick back in; the doctor cautioned that could take another week.

If the aspiration-related stumbling blocks don't resolve by next Wednesday, it is possible that they will do a tracheostomy so Ben can be more mobile, start some PT, and finally get on the road to recovery. But even if they get the physical stuff under control, it may take quite a while to get his mental acuity back, and he's been bed-ridden all month, so he's going to need a lot of physical therapy to regain his strength.

Sorry this missive is so long. Tried pulling lots of strings today in an effort to be given permission to see him, to no avail, but one result was that I had several conversations with various members of his team.

The two common themes that each member circled back to were

1. Ben's remarkable resiliency and

2. the fact that he has received "a young, strong heart."

As part of the regular post-transplant protocol, tomorrow he will be taken to the cath lab for a biopsy of the new heart to assess how it is doing in its new home, a test that will be repeated many times over the next several months.

As the last doctor who spoke with me this evening pointed out, Ben was "extremely" sick before surgery. So the challenge is that he is recovering from much more than "just" a heart transplant.

xoxoxo SAC

A week post-transplant, I spoke with Nurse Beverly at 5:15 a.m. Ben hadn't gotten much sleep, but his arterial blood gases had improved, and the chest tubes had drained off goodly amounts of fluid. "He's looking much better than yesterday," she said.

At noontime, Nurse Brent reported that they'd been able to lower one of the settings on the ventilator and that the blood gases were still looking good. He gave me a heads-up that they'd be calling sometime soon for consent for the first of what would be regular biopsies of the new heart to detect any signs of rejection, and he facilitated a brief Face-Time so that I could lay eyes on Ben and see and hear all the tubes and machines and screens and soft beeps and swishes. Although his eyes were open, there didn't appear to be anybody home.

"Hey, Ben. I know you're too tired to focus, but know that I'm here waiting for you to come back to me. You've got so many people there looking out for you, and so many others out here in the world praying and sending positive thoughts for your recovery. You've got everyone's attention: the doctors, the nurses, our boys, your mother, your sister, my dad, Pete, Dan, and Jon . . .

"I need you to pay attention: right now it's as if you're playing a back game in backgammon and have a couple of men on the bar—but your opponent has got lots of men left on the board yet, and his six-point is open.

"It's time for you to roll double sixes. Right now. Come on, Ben: you can do it."

When the request for consent came at 4:00 p.m., however, it turned out to be for the tracheostomy, which meant the biopsy had been postponed for a day.

Shortly afterward, Dr. Bush called. "I think they're still optimistic."

The word "still" unnerved me, but he continued gently, "This is a roller coaster. You can't get too carried away by the ups or too discouraged by the downs."

But doing a trache so soon after major surgery? It'd only been seven days. "Some people think a trache is a last desperate measure; it's not. Hang in."

The tracheostomy was performed by Dr. Brozzi, the transplant surgeon, who left a message afterward that "surgery went well; he's stable."

Sometimes I'd wake up too early to call the hospital. For distraction, I'd follow what had become my usual practice of sitting on the porch and looking at the stars, or if it was cloudy, I'd play the *New York Times* Spelling Bee game. Or I'd work on some sudokus or KenKen puzzles.

Friday was one of those mornings. I managed to hold off on calling until 4:45 a.m. When I got through to Nurse Beverly again, she told me that Ben had gotten some sleep and his labs looked better. He'd begun to communicate by blinking. He was on low-dosage blood-pressure meds. It looked like a biopsy was on the day's schedule.

At 9:50 a.m., the call came requesting my consent.

"I am Benjamin Cart's wife, Sarah Cart. His birthdate is . . . I understand that you want to do an endomyocardial biopsy to assess any potential signs of rejection of the heart he received on April 16. I give my consent for this procedure."

Afterward, Nurse Marisa arranged for a brief FaceTime so I could see Ben. His ability to interact was about 0.3, and the white tracheostomy dressing at his neck made him look like a priest. But Marisa also checked his chart and said that the overnight dialysis volume was more than a liter, and his chest was still draining a little. While he was too weak even to squeeze her hand, she wanted me to know that he could and would blink on command and answer her questions . . . if he were awake and alert enough.

"The improvements are subtle, but they're there. Hang in. Call back if you want, but don't panic if I don't pick up when the desk forwards you to my phone."

On that afternoon's daily phone call, that week's Dr. Hernandez reported that the orthopedists had no recommendation except to note that Ben's hip would likely require surgery eventually. His white blood count was improving. He was off the blood-pressure vasopressors ("pressers" for short), and the result of his biopsy was a grade of 1R—indicating mild rejection, equivalent to a B+. In addition to an antiviral drug, they'd finally been able to start him on Prograf, the transplant-specific immunosuppressant.

Before getting off her shift, Nurse Marisa facilitated another Face-Time session; this time Ben's cognition had improved to a 0.9.

"Your grandchildren's posters arrived, and he seems to have registered them. They're wonderfully bright and cheerful. We've taped them up so he has something to see other than the bare white walls."

For several days now, my meditation time had been devoted to calling forth that column of healing light so it illuminated the whole hospital campus. I visualized Ben's army of guardian angels surrounding his hospital bed with an all-enveloping miraculous energy. I imagined the angels individually: providing strength to his heart were his father, his paternal grandmother, his maternal grandfather, and one of his best friends from high school. At his head were his paternal grandfather, his aunt, and his maternal grandmother. Elsewhere in the room were my mother, the donor, my brother, my brother-in-law, my stepbrother, and so, so, so many others. I begged them to help Ben find his way back. To all of us. To me.

Friday, April 24
Full day no. 8

Hi, all—

Yesterday's agenda for taking care of Ben changed from what had been outlined on Wednesday.

The surgeon who performed the transplant performed a tracheostomy, and so the first of his weekly endomyocardial biopsies didn't take place until today. Both procedures went well, and the biopsy results were exactly what the doctors were expecting.

Although dialysis continues, his white blood count is improving slowly. His blood gases are better. His blood pressure is good (119/60), and he is breathing on his own occasionally.

Being totally subjective here, on a scale of 1 to 10, yesterday's one FaceTime session merited a 0.02, and I would rate the two we had today at 0.3 and 0.9 respectively.

Yes, all three of those numbers are painfully low, but they represent vast progress over the course of 24 hours.

Part of the improvement is surely attributable to the replacement of the breathing tube with the tracheostomy gear (which makes him vaguely resemble a man of the cloth) . . . and the nurse pointed out that several other leads have been removed from his head and neck. She also reported that he brightened at the arrival of the posters created by Sunny, Courtland, Sander, and Weatherly, which are now taped to the wall where he will be able to see them as his focus improves.

As many of you know, Ben has an uncanny ability to roll double sixes at the most critical moments in backgammon. When I spoke with his night nurse at five o'clock this morning, I asked her to tell him that he needed to start rolling double sixes; when she did, she said there was a trace of a reaction.

During each of today's FaceTimes, I repeated the same thing. Each time there was a hint of some light behind his eyes. Certainly nothing resembling focus or recognition, but a smidgen of curiosity, maybe, at the sound of my voice and the tempting challenge of a good back game.

Maybe tomorrow's phone calls will have the rattling of a dice cup as their soundtrack.

xoxoxo SAC

During a 5:50 a.m. conversation with Nurse Alexa on Saturday morning, she reported that they were slowly weaning Ben off the blood-pressure medications and that she'd been playing music for him—Beatles, mostly. That sounded wonderful to me, and I recommended anything from the *Revolver* album ("Good Day Sunshine," "I'm Only Sleeping," "Yellow Submarine," "Here, There and Everywhere").

Aching to witness visible improvement, a few hours later I tried getting through on the phone with little luck. After I spent ten minutes on hold, the line would roll over to a busy signal. Then it would do it again. When I finally managed to get through, the nurse wasn't free to talk, but she promised to call back. When she did, we got disconnected. On the next try, we agreed to FaceTime in half an hour.

"Oh, what a relief to be able to see both of you! Thank you, Alexa."

"We can't stay on long, but I promise, we will call back before I go off shift."

Ben's response then, and again when we FaceTimed in the late afternoon, wasn't great—0.2 out of ten and then at 5:00 p.m., a 0.5. But at least it felt like there might be something there. Alexa reported that she put *Raiders of the Lost Ark* on for him, and every so often it felt as if he was checking it out.

On Sunday, after that rough three-day stretch in the tomb, during the morning's nurse-facilitated FaceTime, I was amazed when Ben gave a wave, then reached out to hold the iPad himself. An exponential improvement over the previous two days, which themselves had been exponential improvements over Thursday—or at least an improvement over the view I'd had of him on Thursday, full of tubes and wires, mouth agape to accommodate the breathing tube, eyes rolled up into his head and not even half closed.

While Ben's wave buoyed me, the rest of that day was gray and muggy, with too much desk work and not enough focus. Lots of thank-you notes to write and many days' worth of emails and text messages to process. I'd been trying to respond to all in a timely fashion, but whenever it became emotionally exhausting, I'd give up, so lots of caring folks were falling through the cracks.

So many, many thank-yous—for comfort food, cookies and tea loaves, golf-cart cocktails and roadside pep talks, parking-lot blessings, cards and letters and Zoom sessions; all the hospital folks; neighbors' smiles of encouragement and sighs of empathy; waves and hellos and calls of "We're praying for you both"; socially distanced picnic suppers and morning coffee chats, and so much more.

Flipping through my calendar, I had to give thanks that even as *dozens* of events and appointments had been crossed out, canceled because of the pandemic, numerous other entries had replaced them.

CHAPTER 9

To a Galaxy Far, Far
Away and Back Again

April 26, 2020—April 30, 2020

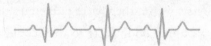

A ll his life, Ben has had vivid dreams and the ability to recall them in great detail later. During the second half of April 2020 and into May, most likely thanks to the miracles of modern pharmacology, his subconscious traveled via wild dreams and hallucinations to worlds far beyond our comprehension, worlds he still recalls keenly.

Routinely, every morning since Ben had arrived at the hospital, the nurses asked him a series of questions to assess his mental status, usually at the same time as they gave him his meds. Typically, that meant they'd ask him to state his name, his birthdate, where he was, the current date (the month was sufficient), and who the president was. Early on, these questions were easy, but as the weeks went by and ICU delirium set in, his brain fast-forwarded from spring to fall to winter, and one morning when a nurse asked him about the president, he accused her of trying to trick him.

"Do you think I don't know about the plane and the shotgun and the assassination? He thought he could act like a hero, but they got him. Or did he just set it up to make it look that way? I think they did get him, but I don't know if they got the vice president too. So does that make the correct answer the Speaker of the House?"

After the transplant, Ben sank deep into a parallel universe where he experienced a complex alternative reality that even novelist Stephen King, master of supernatural fiction, would have found impressive. While some elements appeared to have their genesis in the real world, the origin of the rest will forever remain a mystery.

For starters, Ben was convinced that all the various procedures and operations he was undergoing were happening aboard a plane, with the hospital's blessing.

In this strange new world, there were numerous aircraft where people were harvesting human body parts so they could manufacture sets of twins and perfect babies, and there was an all-encompassing Wi-Fi system that linked each person to every other person. The system would disconnect and turn off automatically if people didn't coordinate "properly." No speaking was allowed, and nobody was recognizable, even to themselves.

There was also a conglomerate of some sort that owned and operated four big nuclear-powered motors at four separate sites around the world. Each location housed one of these massive matching generators and cooling units inside a ginormous glassy building where merchandise was manufactured. A lot of our friends had borrowed money to be able to invest in this conglomerate; proceeds from the sale of an extensive range of goods and countless marketing tie-ins were paying for everything.

One of the merchandise categories was bespoke furniture. One could pick a motif or style as well as the size of a piece, and then the machines would generate it. It appeared to be a criminal operation. There was no need for any insurance or best practices because everyone was making money. The entire situation was probably illegal, but the hospital was looking the other way.

There were also medical machines that could change one's body according to one's specifications. This aspect of the business was based in the ceiling of Ben's room, and high-end mists and sprays enhanced the transformative experience. In this parallel dimension, a few of our closest friends and one nurse were privy to all the details. This narrow circle ensured its exclusivity and resulted in it being exceedingly expensive, although there were also opportunities to buy in, own a share, and recoup one's investment (with one's return dependent on how early one had gotten in on the deal, of course). It was in one's best interests to recruit and retain other investors.

The offerings included plastic surgery, body sculpting, genetic engineering, and more, all performed on private jets linked by computer. Time zones complicated things, as did wireless access. There was also "a water problem" wherein people's bodies would fill with or secrete liquids, which was a giveaway to the illegal goings-on. Making all this especially challenging was that twice each day, the hospital turned off all the Wi-Fi connections. As for the profits, any money the investors made had to be spent in a huge virtual marketplace. Oh, and people routinely employed enormous bodyguards.

Deep in his hallucinatory state, when Ben was given the choice of opting in, staying in, or getting out of his role as an investor, he opted to get out, but he had credit with one good friend, who paid him back. Then everything fell apart when the plane crashed ("but that's a whole other story").

The nearly irresistible element of the potential investment—the most tempting aspect of all—was the opportunity to take part in fabulous hunting and fishing expeditions with amazing tour guides and dogs pursuing mythically large prey. Ben was especially drawn to this because he had befriended an ancient Japanese man who owned the same kind of gun as he did. There were these large boats and the chance to chase after massive fish. The boat's captain would have to shoot at the fish to set the hook. If he did well, over time he could earn enough credit to pay for his gun, enabling him to make a living.

Then for some inexplicable reason, one of the four nuclear units used in merchandise production was turned off. Another unit was damaged by a typhoon, and upon inspection, the authorities uncovered a hidden fiber that had surreptitiously kept the first unit running. When they checked the other three nuclear facilities, they discovered that this same type of fiber had been keeping those running too, prompting a forensic investigation.

As a result, one friend's family life was turned upside down. The family had a wonderful bodyguard, an old Swedish seafaring captain and former wrestler (six feet four, gaunt, a perfect physical specimen) who could secretly absorb all the extra fluid generated during the airborne procedures. If those same procedures were performed on land, the patient could run into a pool or the ocean, but without someone like the Swedish bodyguard, anyone on a plane would be stuck having to deal with all that moisture pouring out of his or her body.

The friend was in a box with a noose, and the family was having to move to the Caribbean because they were about to be arrested as a result of all their illegal activities. Both children in the family were nurses at the clinic. One would come in and chat with Ben from time to time, and the other was having a sex-change operation that involved being shipped via cargo to the US Virgin Islands for the transition, then returned to the United States with a new passport. Because of the business fiasco, the friend and his wife were undergoing plastic surgery so no one would recognize them. In their case, the water problem was especially pronounced, so they needed additional bodies to absorb the extra fluids as the operations progressed, otherwise their suspicious behavior would draw the attention of the authorities.

Another friend had also been involved in the shady business that had both families actively harvesting body parts, so while it was believed that he was shopping with his family at a megamall, he was, in fact, undergoing plastic surgery as well.

Meanwhile (because all this wasn't complicated enough), there was a saleswoman, a friend of Ben's sister, who had figured out how to keep selling shares in the conglomerate and making money for the investors. No attention had been paid to contingencies or depreciations. The saleswoman had enabled an embezzling scheme to which Ben's sister and brother-in-law were party. As a result, the couple now owed us money. Not long after Ben was finally well enough to hold his own phone and make his own calls, he reached out and directed me to get a hold of his sister ASAP. He needed me to explain to her that their scheme had come to light. He also wanted me to set up a payment plan through which they could repay the stolen funds over a series of months. Oh, and by the way, in case I hadn't heard, Ben had Face-Timed with Benjamin and Anna on Benjamin's laptop as they were leaving for their honeymoon (there was no point in trying to explain to him that, with the world still shut down because of COVID, no one was going anywhere).

But well before he was able to use his own phone again, and be disabused of such notions, the hallucinations of his dreamlike state ran amok. Ben believed everyone in our immediate family had scattered and gone into hiding. He thought two of our sons had died because he had been given $1.5 million by the Chinese to compensate him for their deaths and keep him quiet. Then he learned, however, that James and Ashley and the children had been found, William was "safe," and Ted was being kept in a vault in Baltimore.

Meanwhile, civilization was being managed by a multilevel world registry operating beneath the surface of the earth, and survival depended on the food pellets distributed to each "registered life." People became small units. The assumption was that after "the blast," the world had become a giant tundra and all human life had moved underground.

At one point, somehow, Ben figured out who and where I was, yet he thought I didn't know who or where he was. He was waiting for Christmas, because that would be the day he could leave the plane where all his various procedures and operations had taken place, and he could finally make it to the hospital lounge, where I would be waiting for him. He felt that if he could somehow just get into that big room, the one with the high ceiling, we'd be able to communicate with each other via a code that involved blinking when we looked at certain ceiling tiles.

In order for us to be able to spend the holiday together, I was going to have to find and identify him—an especially challenging task since people didn't look like themselves anymore. But unlike the situation on the plane, even though people weren't recognizable to anyone else, they were at least recognizable to themselves. Ben was spending hours scheming to get near me so he could distinguish himself wordlessly, assuming I would know from his mannerisms exactly who he was. If we could recognize each other as husband and wife, we'd be allowed to eat meals together. But apparently, in order for me to get to the lounge area, I had to keep waiting for something, like an advertisement, that would be the ultimate signal, so that even if I'd never been allowed to go to the lounge before, I'd be allowed to go this time. Above all, it was critical that I arrive in time for Christmas.

Recounting all this months later, Ben told me that we did manage to find each other, even though it was for only the briefest moment, and that he wept with happiness.

During Sunday's 5:20 a.m. conversation, the night nurse reported that although Ben had been spared several of the medications overnight, he did have to be sedated because he kept trying to move his arms and legs, an impossibility with all the tubes. His blood pressure was staying "elevated," at 120/68.

Figuring I had little to lose, I dialed back at 8:50 a.m. This was the first time Nurse Michael had been responsible for Ben, but he was game to facilitate a FaceTime session, and oh, it did my soul good.

Ben waved! And he held the iPad and reacted positively to the idea of listening to Billy Joel, Reba McEntire, and maybe watching *Avatar*. While he was far from well, his communication ability had progressed to 2.0. Michael mentioned that the television was on a news channel.

"Oh, please, no—there is nothing in the news that will help his recovery!"

Excited and overestimating the options for entertainment, however, I suggested instead that if he could watch other movies besides *Raiders of the Lost Ark*—perhaps some musicals, *Little Shop of Horrors*, or a real oldie like *Guys and Dolls*—those would help reawaken Ben's psyche. Or if television proved too burdensome, music alone would be great. Country, Queen, or Elton John would make Ben happy.

Relieved and grateful for the tremendous, albeit incremental, progress of the previous thirty-six hours, yet ever mindful that Ben still had a long fight ahead, I now had the luxury of worrying about what might happen next.

His recovery needed to span a broad spectrum, from physical to mental. Who would assess his executive function and when? Was there a battle plan for moving forward? And how long would the hospital remain committed to standing by Ben's side?

During the doctor's midafternoon phone update, I heard that he'd been well enough for a physical therapy evaluation of his range of motion, done with no sedation. No vasopressors were needed to keep his blood pressure up. These were tremendous milestones. I didn't want to ask but had to: "At what point do you kick him out of the SICU to some sort of critical-care rehab?"

"That won't happen. He won't go to rehab until he has progressed well enough for it to help him further."

That was the moment I realized they'd never knowingly ask us to perform without a net.

By now, our FaceTime sessions had lengthened to forty-five to sixty seconds, about the limit of what Ben could tolerate before giving in to exhaustion, but by Sunday afternoon's call, during which he merited a full 2.5, he was nodding or shaking his head in response to yes-or-no questions. And at the end, he mouthed "Goodbye" and put his hand to his lips.

My eyes welled up as I hit the button to disconnect. It had been a long week, from his being extubated and giddy to crashing, but maybe I could finally begin to believe he might possibly be on his way back to me.

Sunday, April 26
Full day no. 10

Hi, all—

Yesterday brought no significant changes in Ben's status or awareness, so this morning when the nurse agreed to facilitate the first of our twice-daily FaceTime sessions, I nearly dropped my phone when Ben slowly but definitely waved.

The nurse then let him hold the iPad briefly as I asked him some basic questions, each eliciting a slow nod or shake of his head. The nurse took the iPad back when Ben was obviously spent from the effort.

By the end of call no. 2, six hours later, Ben was slightly more purposeful in the shaking or nodding his head in response to simple questions ("Would you like them to play Billy Joel for you?"), and although again he tired easily, he mouthed "Goodbye" when he was ready to give the iPad back to the nurse. Then he put his hand to his lips: when the nurse asked if he was blowing a kiss, he nodded his head yes.

The slow dialysis continues, but he was only mildly sedated overnight. His blood pressure is holding steady (120/68), and he had some range-of-motion physical therapy today.

So. Baby steps, but a lot of them in the right direction in just the past 24 hours and hugely uplifting.

Giving thanks: for the doctors' continued close attention to too many details to list, for the nurses' unending TLC and patience, for Ben's resilience, for miracles. And for all of you and the many friends from all parts of his and our lives who are thinking of him, praying for him, pulling for him.

xoxoxo SAC

By Monday's late morning FaceTime, during which the nurse explained that dialysis would likely be more effective now that some of Ben's medications had been reduced, he was tired but awake and aware throughout the call, vastly different from the out-of-it state of the previous eight days. And he had slept all the way through the night before.

Dr. Hernandez called that afternoon, optimistic because, as he said, everything looked good. "We're experimenting with stopping dialysis to see if that helps Ben's kidneys kick back on. To do that, we'll go with more intermittent dialysis and see what happens." He observed, just as I had noticed that morning, that "Ben is both more with it and more fatigued. The physical therapy team came by, and he engaged in more range-of-motion activities, and he's tolerating the CPAP and oxycodone."

And he advised, "Whenever you have a chance to FaceTime with Ben, encourage him to move and do what you can to cheer him up."

I gave it my best shot during our late afternoon session, and Ben sort of smiled, but he was spent.

Tuesday morning, the night nurse, Stacy, reported that Ben was breathing on his own without assistance from the ventilator. No sedation; no vasopressors. And he was producing small amounts of urine. He'd also watched television until 2:00 a.m.

"Was he really watching, or was it just on?"

"Oh, no. I'd say he was paying attention, even if he didn't necessarily grasp what was happening."

Although I'd never been a fan of Ben's middle-of-the-night television habits, at that moment I was thrilled to hear he was resuming them.

Later in the day, the team added a Passy Muir valve to his tracheostomy so he could talk, although when we FaceTimed midafternoon, he was distracted, uncharacteristically grumpy, and unwilling to engage with me. As soon as the doctors walked in, mid–phone call, and asked how he was, however, he perked right up for them: "I'm in great spirits!"

Dr. Hernandez reported that the next biopsy was scheduled for Friday, May 1.

At the end of the day, I took a call from a technician needing consent to change Ben's dialysis setup from CVVHD (continuous veno-venous hemodialysis) to TDC (temporary dialysis catheter). The switch would have to happen under sedation: radiology would do so via his jugular, using ultrasound. There would be small incisions in his neck and chest, along with antibiotics. The risks, while minimal, included the possibility of infection.

"My name is Sarah Cart. I am the wife of Benjamin Cart . . ."

Consent granted.

Tuesday, April 28
Full day no. 12

Hi, all—

This morning a little valve was added to Ben's tracheostomy gear enabling him to speak, and although we weren't able to talk much, he sounds just like himself, if a bit slow and still very confused.

He wanted to know where I was and when I'm going to come pick him up. After saying "I'm in the kitchen," I wasn't sure what to say next, not wanting to disappoint . . .

But then I remembered that while I was out walking yesterday, a black racer had skirted safely across a two-lane road immediately in front of me, and I'd thought, "Ben will be happy to hear about that." Well, he was. And he was happy to hear that a redstart has been flitting about in the bushes just outside the front door.

Tomorrow, Ben's temporary dialysis catheter (which goes into his neck and via which they've been handling his slow dialysis) will be replaced with a tunnel one in his chest (more stable, and perhaps enabling him to be a bit mobile). Then they will try having the dialysis be intermittent rather than constant and see how his kidneys respond.

His next regularly scheduled endomyocardial biopsy will be on Friday. A bit of a tortoise day—giving thanks for slow and steady progress.

xoxoxo SAC

On day 14 of his new heart, Ben woke after a restless night (probably because he had slept so much the day before) to declare during our Face-Time session that he was "Ben Cart one two three four."

I wasn't sure what he meant, but he showed the most energy he'd had in more than ten days.

Thursday, April 30
Full day no. 14

Hi, all—

Not much new to report. Ben continues to make slow progress in the right direction. The doctors remain pleased. But because he's able to communicate better, the extent of his confusion is more evident when we talk.

This morning, he'd just stirred from a dream that he was sleeping comfortably in the back of a pickup truck that had brought him home, then was disappointed to find he was still in the hospital. Later, as we FaceTimed, he was noticeably sad because he wants to be home but doesn't know the way. Savvy showed up next to me on cue, however, to cheer him up a bit.

And yet just two weeks ago, he got a new heart, and one week ago was the day our FaceTime session rated 0.02 on a scale of 1 to 10. Today he woke up having dreamed he slept comfortably, and *we talked*. The simplest of conversations, but conversation nonetheless.

An Ohio friend catching up on all the details of the past month summarized it yesterday as "slow but steady progress, which is wonderful. He is so deconditioned—and OF COURSE he also has a hip fracture (why not?!). It sounds like he ended up in the right place just in time—what wonderful staff!"

Tying up one loose end from last week's culture tests: they never grew anything, and looking forward, he heads in for endomyocardial biopsy no. 2 tomorrow.

xoxo SAC

For me, writing these communiques served several purposes. Each one was a memo from the front lines, crafted to be loving and true, and the process of writing them helped me sort and settle my head and heart, even on those days when sorting and settling either felt impossible.

With every single report, I pounded a stake in the ground: "Here's how far we've come. The progress may be slow, but this is what it looks like."

And so far, the emails had also served to keep everyone on the same page and safeguard my emotional resources, even as I was only now coming to appreciate that in the fog of war, Ben and I were each slogging across separate battlefronts.

CHAPTER 10

Reemergence

April 30, 2020—May 12, 2020

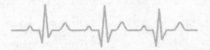

At the clinic, Ben was beginning to reengage with the world and was on the cusp of making significant progress, but his brain was a mess from disuse and drugs and weeks of hallucinatory dreams, and his body was ravaged. Bedridden; stifled by the ventilator; waiting for his kidneys to kick back in; still full of IVs, drainage tubes, and a urinary catheter; dependent on nurses to charge his hearing aids and insert them for him so he could understand what they were saying; exasperated by his glasses' outdated prescription; wishing someone could find the time to trim his fingernails—he was frustrated, short-tempered, and uncharacteristically emotional.

On the home front, I was doing all I could to advocate on his behalf from a distance, but I continued to wrestle with unreliable cell coverage in our new quarters. It was complicating my interactions (or lack thereof) with the nurses and doctors and undermining my faith that they'd be able to reach me instantly in the event of an emergency. If I left a message for them, I would ask that they ring the landline because I felt I could trust it more, but then I'd have to stay home to wait for their call. If I was at the house and they happened to dial my cell number—because that was the number listed first on Ben's chart—the call would go straight to voice mail.

I had not been able to muster the energy until now to contact our wireless network operator, knowing that the best-case scenario if I tried to arrange for more consistent coverage would likely involve hours on hold, and I wasn't wrong. A five-hour session late Thursday, with an incredibly patient tech consultant, failed to get the correct settings working, much to his surprise. We agreed to call it a night and resigned, discouraged and exhausted, I fell asleep fully clothed on top of my bed, only to wake at 4:00 a.m. when Savvy, whom I'd accidentally left outside for the duration, woke me by scratching at the door.

When I picked up my phone, however, I could see deep in the settings that it was finally working properly! Bless the tech: he'd kept at it even after I'd given up.

Meanwhile, there were the day-to-day responsibilities of being a homeowner, which included more frequent dealings with plumbers, electricians, and carpenters than usual as the settling-in process after the move continued. COVID protocols (and, early on, Savvy's fleas) made every task more complicated.

But we'd made it to May—a new month. Time to give thanks for the chance to begin again.

The hospital's call for consent to conduct Ben's second post-op biopsy came at 7:30 a.m. Friday, and from the moment my cell rang all the way through the conversation with the nurses, the exchange went just as it was supposed to, without any surprises or delays—a blessing and milestone. After the usual statement of identification and confirmation of Ben's birthdate, I assented to their doing an endomyocardial biopsy to assess any potential signs of rejection.

Thanks to Ben's nurses, he and I FaceTimed later that morning, and the doctors stopped in to tell us that, after thirty-five days, there was a chance he'd move out of the SICU over the weekend.

Then in the afternoon, Ben placed his first phone call *on his own* to our landline, a number he hadn't been sure of a couple of weeks ago. He was wildly confused, all over the place with news, plans, and instructions. He reported that he'd "watched a different movie last night," then warned me that I needed to "demand the money back that my sister is embezzling from us" and revealed that "the machinery that shrink-wraps the brown furniture isn't working." He wanted to know what I was doing about getting him out of the hospital, and finally, he demanded that I run some nonsensical errands and track down some nonexistent phone messages. I wanted to celebrate a step forward, but I worried this conversation marked a major step backward.

That night, while I was on a Zoom call catching up with our boys, Ben called his mother. She was ecstatic and emailed everyone in her address book immediately afterward, saying that he sounded strong and not confused at all. She also mentioned that he told her he'd be moving out of the SICU first thing the next morning.

Saturday was tough. My mother-in-law's sharing of Ben's apparent good news meant I had an inbox full of congratulations and expectations to be tempered as quickly and gently as possible.

And while I was busy responding to those messages on my laptop from Ben's desk, I could see on his computer that Ben was broadening his horizons, signing into his email account for the first time since late March. It wasn't long before an email from his account landed in mine.

SUBJECT: *I m m mmnot trsffu trsftu yo yo fo fonfo*

MESSAGE: No info on Hossam you know it takes a long time.

Wondering what in the world he was trying to convey, I called his phone. Good news: he answered.

Bad news: I couldn't make sense of all he had to say, and he said a lot.

"My sister and her husband's embezzling happened while I was in the hospital last summer, so we didn't collect from them. There was a storm. It's the same amount of money as is being used for the green table that we haven't been paid for. You need to ask them to pay it back. It would be great to have that in our account moving forward."

"I had some soup yesterday; hoping to have a banana today."

"My mission is to have somebody arrive with food for you and your pet."

I wondered if he meant Savvy or if he was remembering catching John Wick six weeks earlier.

"Oh, and by the way, how's your dad?"

I replied, "He's well. He asks about you every day, and—"

"I've got a bird here on the lightbulb."

I asked, "What kind?"

"We'll have to figure him out . . . Black."

"Also, it would be good to come to terms with my sister and brother-in-law to determine how much they have to pay us for the nuclear stuff."

"Your job is to log on to the insurance website so that we can reimburse Mark for what the company's paying."

I was reeling, and he wasn't done.

At last, he announced he needed to hang up, but offered, "Let's FaceTime again at four; call me."

Saturday, May 2
Full day no. 16

Hi, all—

No word yet on the results of yesterday's endomyocardial biopsy, but a few hours after the procedure was completed, the doctors stopped in to tell Ben he might move out of the SICU to a "regular room" today, an awesome step in the right direction. The reality, however, is that in order for that to happen, they need to write up the orders *and* a room for him to move into needs to be available. As of this writing (3:00 p.m.), both those steps remain to be taken.

And while he is better able to talk and can sound strong and coherent, his confusion continues. In an hourlong noontime conversation, he was deeply concerned that we are being embezzled by someone close to us, and he was encouraging me to get after that situation and ask for the money to be returned.

Yet in the midst of the muddle, he injected two absolutely timely comments, one inquiring after somebody else's health and the other about an insurance premium that comes due at the beginning of each month.

So. Wonderful progress with some bizarre weirdness on the side. Hopefully he will be in a new room soon, and once away from the busyness of the SICU, his head will clear more quickly and completely.

xoxoxo SAC

While I couldn't follow any of Ben's other instructions, at least I could make the 4:00 p.m. call, though he aborted that conversation quickly. "Not interested in talking right now but say hi to Savvy Dabby Doo for me!"

Click.

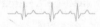

Six months earlier, we had marked Saturday, May 2, on our calendars as the date our family would gather outside Nashville to be with youngest son, Benjamin, and his fiancée, Anna, as they exchanged wedding vows. But when the pandemic arrived, they'd decided to postpone the event for a year. Still, though, when the day arrived, they determined to go ahead despite everything, and their minister agreed that they could meet in her backyard that afternoon with the bride's kitten, Pippa, serving as flower girl and the groom's pup, Link, the wonder mutt–mystery hound, standing up as best man.

Within the hour, they called me to share the news, and I immediately called the nurses' station. It took a moment for the mentally exhausted nurse who answered to understand what I was asking her to share with Ben, but as soon as she did, I could hear her announce it to all the staff around her desk, and they whooped with joy.

Bless the newlyweds—the two of them could have simply said, "Nope, not doing this now. Too complicated," but instead they had carried out an inspiring act of faith in the future even as the daily news was so dark and disheartening and, in that act, uplifted all of us across the miles.

Shortly thereafter, Ben called in tears, absolutely devastated not to be able to figure out how to reach the bride and groom.

"Tell them I love them very much." He hung up.

I called Benjamin, who in turn called his father a few minutes later, then got back to me. "Dad was very happy, although he doesn't understand that we're sheltering in place in Tennessee. He thinks we're in Bermuda on our honeymoon."

Sunday proved long and tough too. Early on, Nurse Danielle told me that Ben had a restless night and was expressing deep frustration at not having been moved into a new room, but she advised me not to push for that. I might not be hearing from the doctors as often as I'd like, but so long as he was in the SICU, he'd be tracked constantly, which was the more important thing at the moment. By the time I went to bed that night, I would gain a much deeper appreciation for that wisdom.

Danielle arranged for a midday FaceTime, and I was thrilled to see Ben in a chair, out of bed for the first time in weeks, but we had to hang up almost immediately because the doctors arrived just then for rounds.

A couple of hours later, the doctor called, full of news. Friday's biopsy had shown evidence of moderate rejection, giving Ben a grade of 2R, so he was just finishing up forty-eight hours of high-dose steroids.

I was alarmed at the news. An echocardiogram, however, showed that the left and right sides of the heart were performing normally. He was swallowing well and was now clear of C. diff—

"Wait: what's C. diff?"

"*Clostridium difficile*, a type of bacterium that can cause colitis and inflammation of the colon. The infection isn't unusual, given how long he's been in the hospital, his weakened immune system, and the kidney issues."

The doctor continued: despite Ben's petitioning hard, the doctors didn't want to move him out of the SICU over the weekend. He'd been off the ventilator for three days and hadn't needed any blood-pressure medications. He did produce some urine two nights ago.

I knew all this was fabulous progress, but dammit, I was frustrated at the bits that were news: the steroids, the gut issue, the (slight) kidney progress.

Lastly, the next biopsy should happen on Friday or so.

Within the hour, Ben called to say he was in a new room. I hated not believing him, but there was no way that could be true, was there?

Since one of my day-to-day challenges was responding to friends and family members who were wondering whether the cards and packages they'd sent to Ben at the hospital had been received, I asked Ben if he'd gotten any mail.

"Yes. I got a rock, like Charlie Brown, from Cedric."

I didn't know how to respond, but I didn't need to, because he kept right on going. "I'm having all kinds of problems with my phone, so I'm turning off lots of apps, but at least it's plugged in."

I was flummoxed, as confused as he was. Who knew what he might do if he got deep into his phone's settings? I just hoped that whatever he did would prove reversible.

He also explained they'd had to use a crane to get him out of bed and into the chair. "That was one of Daddy's last rides; it was awful."

"The view of the birds is different. I want to come home. I want to be able to look outside to see the birds and the sunset."

And then he was done. Click.

Two hours later, I received a phone call from casual, but kind and loving, acquaintances whose phone number happened to fall alphabetically right after mine in Ben's contacts. They'd received a call from him, during which he explained that he was "trying really hard to get to the next level." Ugh.

As the evening continued, I heard from his sister, who'd heard from him around eight, and then Jon reached out, having received several texts, two of which also came to me.

"I have asked to be re-enstated [sic] under jon goals of church and orange jello 😎" and "Cedric ok wt it. Ulcers gone." Ugh. Ugh. And ugh again.

Jon took the opportunity to suggest that I investigate the location of dialysis facilities in the Keys and explained that at Hartford, heart transplant patients have one year of "stay-close follow-up" appointments. Sensing that I was war-weary, at the end of our conversation he reassured me, "The 2R grade simply means his body is mounting a response. That's a good sign."

Then one of Ben's cardiologists called around 9:00 p.m. to be sure I felt caught up. He'd seen a message that I'd asked for the biopsy results, but no note that the resident physician had been in touch. He confirmed that Ben had had a restless night from Saturday into Sunday, then shared his observation that Ben was experiencing "some confusion." I asked what the chances of his being moved to a regular room the next day were.

"Zero, although the room he's in right now can be re-rated so as not to be considered SICU any longer."

I remembered Nurse Danielle's advice from that morning—not to push for the move. "Please don't do that on my account or on Ben's. He's so wonky right now; I'd prefer the constant attention that comes with being in the SICU."

Sunday night's sleep was my worst in more than two months as I mulled over Ben's state of mind and his loose-cannon behavior. In addition to randomly reaching out via phone or text to simply state that he was "working to get to the next level," he would sometimes go on about "people sneaking around down there" and "the time in the back of the store when all that wild shit was going on."

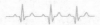

It had been a rough weekend, yes, but in all reality I knew I was well supported. I received expressions of support and encouragement daily, was able to go on long walks and out for socially distanced cocktails and meals, and would then come home to Zoom across the miles with the family and friends who were farther afield.

Every couple of weeks since shortly after the pandemic was declared, seventeen women with whom I'd shared housing during our first year of college had been invited to gather via Zoom. Sometimes only six or seven of us could make it, but more often, we'd show up a dozen or more strong. And every few weeks, I'd Zoom with the crew that had begun as Ben's college roommates and grown to include their wives: Dan and Hitomi, Pete and Jillian, Jon and Carrie. All those friendships were keeping me afloat.

First thing Monday, I wrote myself a note: "The healing power of awareness: remember where he is and why."

Knowing that Ben might call at any time to inquire whether any progress had been made regarding moving him into a new room or discharging him from the hospital or sending him home, I also drafted a list of "stuff to work on before coming home." None of it would be easy to say to him, but at least I had it at my fingertips.

- For your best recovery and health moving forward, you need to be stronger—not just your heart but also your legs and lungs.
- You need to be sleeping regular hours.
- You need to be able to eat real food.
- You need to be able to use the bathroom.
- You need to be able to get around.
- You need to be able to use your iPad.

Plus there were the undeniable mechanical issues, including his ongoing intermittent dialysis, the ventilator, and the CPAP machine. And those were just the ones I knew about.

Then I received a healthy nudge via text from one of my college roommates: "Have your on-a-scale-of-1-to-10 communications with Ben made it to whole numbers yet?"

She was spot-on. We had come miles over the course of one week (0.9 all the way to 4.0). I needed to step back to see the whole forest. Yes, we'd wandered deep into thickets and thorns, but too, there was miraculous progress.

With the new week, I took up the challenge of tracking down the gifts people had sent directly to Ben at the hospital, which was only possible if the senders mentioned having done so. Thanks to some detective work by the hospital operator, I was able to speak with two members of the materials management staff—CeeCee and her boss, Mike—who, overworked as they were, were amazingly gracious and willing to help, so long as I could provide details: vendor, date ordered or sent, shipping company, tracking number. Vendors were having pandemic issues too. Many were short-staffed and cutting expenses by not sending things overnight or priority.

While Ben's mother was particularly distraught because she hadn't received a thank-you from the nurses and doctors to whom she'd sent a huge box of chocolates, his college roommates were hoping the Wi-Fi photo frame they'd sent Ben had safely arrived. It was already full of images recorded over the course of four fun-filled decades of friendship, and able to receive more photos if it were properly plugged in. The aim was to engage his brain, awaken his memories, and help ground him. I prayed they were right. The tracking number showed it had been delivered on April 30, and once I'd armed CeeCee with that information, she promised to complete the mission, although she cautioned that with the mailroom backlog, it might take until the end of the week.

In the middle of Monday morning, Ben called to explain that, like me, he was working on a list, at the top of which was his biggest concern:

"Get Sarah and Jon (working with Cedric) to manage step-down." He informed me that he'd already consulted Jon about getting into step-down so he could, as he said, "process my own food and water and PT." And he continued to share: he was having some ginger ale. No pee. Hoping to use his own bowels today.

Next item: "Figure that dream out. Must have been the Hammonds [Jon and Carrie] or Depews [business partner Mark and his wife, Brenda] in the back of the store. Lots of people sneaking around down there. [This was becoming a common refrain.] Bad stuff. Happy to be out of that room, but we may have to go back there." (Nurse Miguel had already confirmed for me earlier that Ben was still in the same hospital room, which remained rated SICU.)

Tuesday, Ben was in complete loose-cannon mode, beginning with a call to our oldest son, James, at 6:30 a.m. to explain that a young man, a close family friend, had undergone surgery and was now female, but his family wasn't ready to tell anyone. He also asked, in the midst of several non sequiturs, "How's your bunker?"

Reports of similarly bizarre calls to others came in over the next several hours, including one to me. He was positive that he would be on his way back to me within twenty-four hours. He also reported that he "got George Bush on my side for the breakout" (obviously a confused reference to Dr. Bush). Then he asked urgently, "What do we have going on at home?"

And he shifted quickly to make a few things clear: "I'm going to need a hospital bed, a wheelchair, a walker, and a recliner, plus a caregiver to take me to and from the master bathroom toilet."

Finally, he commanded, "Call the hospital social worker right now to determine what's going on."

Near the end of the business day, I put in a panicky call to the hospital social worker, who explained that when Ben talked about step-down, he was referring to something real—i.e., cardiac rehab—but she advised me to tell all family members and friends that "they should run anything Ben tells them by you before they decide it's true."

In the meantime, Tuesday also saw Ben downgraded from SICU status, even as the team was still waiting for a bed in the IMCU (intermediate care unit). He also received some physical therapy. And the close watch on his ability to produce urine continued (if there were none, he'd have dialysis on Wednesday).

The hip surgeon's office weighed in as well: "No question Ben needs surgery. Timing-wise, it will likely be around three weeks after his discharge to home from rehab."

Tuesday, May 5
Full day no. 19

Hi, all—

Quick report: while Ben is still in the same room, his status has been changed, and if a room in the IMCU (intermediate care unit) opens up, they might move him.

All numbers are moving in the right direction, although his kidneys are still on hold.

His confusion rises up in weird ways: texts sent at 3:00 a.m. and a phone call or two made at 6:30 a.m.

As the social worker explained when I called to verify some of the things he told me this afternoon, "Tell your family and friends that they should run anything he says by you before they decide that it's true."

But it's great to have him telling stories!

xoxoxo SAC

As Wednesday dawned, his nurses were touting the progress of his kidneys ("He peed twice last night!"), and I was panicky again. As much as I missed him and ached to see him, touch him, hug him, kiss him on the forehead, and hold his hands, I did not want him home unless he could be safe and properly cared for.

I needed to know more about this mysterious cardiac rehab: Where? When? How long?

Would there be any training or instruction for me? Ben could not come home and sit at his computer thinking he was going to pay bills or settle insurance claims in his current condition, and I was not prepared to turn myself into the head of our own personal nanny state, supervising his every move 24-7. Was I going to have to lock his office door to keep him out of there?

Talking with Ben in the middle of the afternoon only stressed me more, and the conversation didn't end well. He explained, "Susan, the educational nurse, talked with me last night and told me they are releasing me. I have all my personal stuff, so I can leave as soon as you get here."

Oh, dear. Oh, no.

Perhaps he hadn't been wearing his hearing aids, or he had been and he just misheard. Or perhaps he was delusional. But it was clear to me: Ben believed at the core of his being that he was "on his way back to me."

Today.

Logic and reality were absent. I desperately missed the rational Ben, who overthought things and considered every angle and would have insisted on teaching me "Russian grammar" when all I wanted was a simple answer to a straightforward question. Even the ten-year-old-boy version of him, with little capacity for long-range planning, remembering details, or considering consequences—the Ben he'd been four months earlier—would have been preferable to this.

"Ben, you're not coming home today. You can't. I love you and I've missed you terribly, and I can't wait to see you, but you're not ready. I'm not ready. You still have a feeding tube, and we don't know anything about dialysis. Even if it were possible to get all the right furniture and equipment and home health care in place this afternoon, we would not be able to do this. I'm sorry."

He hung up on me. My stomach ached. I felt like I'd just deserted a desperately homesick child at summer camp.

Shortly thereafter, I spoke with Nurse Jennifer, who said they would be releasing Ben to the IMCU, room 413, and noted that she had explained to him that it would be "one step closer to getting home." She also said she'd fielded a call from his mother about the chocolates that had yet to arrive.

It was fascinating how quickly things that were novel not long before had become routine—as well as how quickly new novel details raced at me.

Example: the next day, Thursday, another heart biopsy—routine. News of bedsores—novel and curious. The size of the vent for his trache downsized from 8 to 6—routine. Capping it for a couple of days to see how he tolerates the development—novel. A couple of liters of fluid removed via dialysis—routine. A reference to his incontinence—novel. X-ray reports on his chart regarding degenerative issues at his shoulders and in his spine—novel . . . and terrifying.

All that came from Ben's nurses; I hadn't heard from any doctors since the previous weekend.

But that Thursday was also one of my toughest days yet for a reason that was novel for *me*: Ben refused my calls, a consequence of my being the "but you can't possibly be ready to come home yet" messenger. I'd been dismissed.

When we did finally speak on Friday, Ben sounded so depressed, so *not* himself, that I wondered if I needed to get him a private-duty nurse. I asked him if maybe he should be talking with someone.

He snapped, "Won't make me happy to talk to someone."

Then, as if he were about to cry, "The nurses throw me around." Quietly: "It's different from the SICU; they lie."

I offered a gentle reminder that he was in a hospital, not a hotel.

He responded angrily, "Susan [the educational nurse] gave us the material about how to be discharged," then demanded, "Get me discharged!"

Talking with his nurse at 8:30 a.m. on Friday brought more novel news: Ben had a collapsed lung. At the mundane end of the spectrum, however, she told me that he was already up and sitting in a chair, complaining of pain in his left leg—not a surprise with his broken left hip and his having begun physical therapy.

I was deeply frustrated and hurting on his behalf—and feeling terribly out of the loop, having not heard from any doctors since Sunday. *So* many questions.

Somehow I managed to get through to the cardiothoracic surgeon's administrator, who was able to provide a wealth of answers. With the trache vent size down to 6 from 8, the next step would be to close it. The bedsores? Being addressed. Heart incision looking good. In the last two days, he'd started voiding well. The reason he was finding it hard to talk was because he still had the feeding tube; that would be reevaluated next week.

On Saturday, Ben called at 7:15 a.m. "They're mean to me. There's no hot water. They won't let me use the bathroom. The service is awful. I will pay any amount of money to be someplace else. Get me out of here."

Despite my best efforts to be empathetic, it didn't translate. In frustration, he declared, "I'll have the doctors call you as soon as they come in." Then he hung up on me. Again.

Just after lunch, the nurse called with the doctors' report: two pleural tubes remained, still set at "suction" for a few more days, which meant the slightly collapsed lung was improving by the hour. For now, the staff's priorities for Ben were (1) air, (2) heart, and (3) broken bones. Yes, she used the plural: Was something more than the hip fractured?

I tried to call Ben twice more that afternoon, but he wasn't happy and didn't want to talk with me. That he did talk with William and Ted, our middle sons, however, made me feel a little better. At least he might let them try to lift his spirits.

Ben Reflects

As one of my sons, William, watched from afar during my most difficult days in the hospital, when I was really failing, he later said that my ordeal reminded him of his beloved paternal grandfather's death, in 2015. He told me how hard my situation was for him. Sometimes, especially when he was doing the things we frequently did together, such as hunting, fishing, casting, and canoeing—things I taught him how to do—my not being there was difficult for him. So many sons don't get to be buddies with their dads. But we were buddies. So he didn't want to face up to losing me.

As my condition worsened, William came into a sense of acceptance about the possibility of my death. When I recovered, though, he became oddly angry. He felt he had disrupted his life: he'd overcome his fear and ventured into the difficult world of being there for his dying father as best he could despite the distance. He was kind of at peace with my not ever coming out of the hospital. He was as ready as he could be for me to die.

And then, as in that famous Monty Python scene, I came through and said, "I'm not dead yet!" He was like, "Well, why did you put me through this?" He wasn't sure if he was angry at me or angry at himself, but he thought, "You were supposed to die. I stored up my memories and was working on being at peace with it. And suddenly you're back."

He felt guilty about feeling this way: "What's wrong with me? How can I be angry about a miracle?" But that was only a phase. And he's over his anger and back to being incredibly grateful that I'm here.

William Reflects

There is no standard playbook for death, at least in my mind. The weirdest thing was how angry I was when my father got better. I spent so much time and effort and love making sure I was with him when he was sick. Then one day we get a call and find out he's receiving a heart transplant. Then we get another call and find out he's improving. Then we get more calls and find out he's actually getting totally better.

I didn't know how to cope with it. It was not a conscious choice at all. I am embarrassed by it, but I was angry. I felt like I needed space from him and Mom for a little while, and I wish that had not been the case. I wish I had found more gratitude and balance earlier on.

Saturday, May 9
Full day no. 23

Hi, all—

While parts of Ben's week have been terribly frustrating for him, his progress has been substantial.

A room did open up in intermediate care on Wednesday.

Unfortunately, as they packed everything up, someone explained to him that "it is a first step toward your going home." Ben, however, only heard the end of that sentence, which he interpreted as "You're going home," and was then desperately disappointed.

But his third endomyocardial biopsy was Thursday, and the results were perfect.

And while his kidneys still have a ways to go, they are kicking back in.

Plus he's getting physical therapy several times a day. The tubes in his trachea are getting progressively smaller, and he's being allowed some real food (applesauce, Jell-O, and thick soups), so after the weekend, his need for the feeding tube will be reevaluated.

While he is noticeably more coherent, he is still a bit confused and can be terribly moody, so he doesn't feel up to much communication with the outside world yet and is not "with it" enough to access his emails or texts regularly.

But he's making *huge* strides.

No time frame for the next step or even specifics re: what that will be (although the phrase "cardiac rehab" has been uttered in very general terms), and the orthopedic surgeon would like to operate on Ben's fractured left hip "a few weeks" after he gets home.

Yet in the scheme of things, these are wonderful problems to have.

xoxoxo SAC

When I spoke with a nurse first thing Mother's Day morning, Ben was already washed up and sitting in a chair, having had pancakes and coffee for breakfast after "a good night."

But she then revealed that the doctors were discussing the possibility that Ben had vascular dementia—like "ICU delirium," another thing one should not google.

Ben and I FaceTimed midafternoon, and while he obsessed over "ten steps" regarding his next move and rehab choices, I obsessed about the mechanics of his homecoming, from his being discharged during COVID with a broken hip (and possibly more—no one had confirmed or denied the previous reference to more than one fracture) to countless other details. I needed the doctors to explain Ben's status, the hurdles that remained, and the types of things they expected to happen between now and his discharge. (To rehab? And to home?) What dangers still lay ahead?

Monday morning's report from Nurse Mala was that he'd had lots of bad dreams in the night and as a result was quite lethargic, but when he was awake, he was worrying and fretting. A lot. During one of those spells, he called and urged me to track down Social Worker Jacqueline because "she'll have answers."

Nurse Mala was scheduled to be with him each morning for several days, which eased his confusion somewhat. First thing Tuesday, she told me about an avalanche of progress: his hair had been washed; dialysis was done; the feeding tube was gone; he had no edema; only one chest tube remained. His diet had been upgraded, and he appeared to be tolerating real food. Also, soon I would hear from a nutritionist who would be putting together a packet of heart-healthy dietary information. The speech pathologist would be evaluating his trache later that morning and probably would "red cap" it in anticipation of its removal in a couple of days. And the social worker would be reaching out tomorrow or the day after with specifics regarding rehab.

However, she also explained that the bedsores first mentioned the previous Thursday had merged into one large pressure ulcer at his lower back, which was going to require care and attention for some time.

The message was clear: it had taken an army of medical personnel and support staff to get Ben to this point, and soon that army would be handing his care over to me. Me. Just that: me.

So my notes needed to be precise—like these, which I took while on the phone with the nutritionist:

- The goals: gain strength, muscle, weight.
- Maintain a low-sodium diet (less than 1,200 mg/day).
- For at least twelve months:
  — Food safety is paramount; therefore, eggs and meat should always be well done, no exceptions.
  — Any uneaten foods that might reappear as leftovers should be immediately refrigerated.
  — *Nothing* raw is permitted (sushi, caviar, smoked salmon, soft cheeses, honey, not even sunny-side-up eggs with a runny yolk) (Exception: veggies . . . see below)
- *No* oysters *ever again.*
- Lead with veggies—raw ones are allowed, but ONLY at home (i.e., no restaurant salads).

- Pastas are to be sides rather than mains.
- Proteins are to be defrosted in the fridge, not on the countertop.
- Fridge must be cleaned out now, discarding anything that is expired or that Ben shouldn't have.

Yet again it had been days since I'd had any word from the doctors, despite numerous calls and messages left at the ICMU, and I was becoming disturbingly short-tempered with Ben, finding it increasingly challenging to remain patient with his confusion and loose-cannon episodes while I was serving as his proxy to the outside world. What's more, I had precious little patience for my own roller-coaster moods and feelings—not to mention my frustration over how much or how little I was able to accomplish as each day went by.

I was grateful to his nurses for telling me what they could, but they were constricted, both legally and by the stressful, COVID-magnified load of their daily jobs. Yes, I could read Ben's test results in his online chart, but without a professional to interpret them for me, I was lost, frustrated by my ignorance. How was I supposed to advocate from a void for his best outcomes and care for him if and when we finally managed to get him home?

CHAPTER 11

Marathon Training

May 13, 2020—June 3, 2020

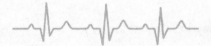

Then at last, one drop at a time, clear answers to my questions began to trickle down—a dribble at first, then a flood.

On Wednesday, Social Worker Beatrice reached out. She told me that a referral had been sent to one of the Memorial Healthcare System's facilities, in Hollywood, next to Fort Lauderdale. The rehab staff was intimately familiar with transplant protocols, including the mechanics of getting Ben back to the hospital for his frequent required follow-up tests, biopsies, and more. She thought perhaps the social workers there might let me visit because they'd have to train me too, and those personnel would make the arrangements for home health care and any equipment that might be needed.

A couple of hours later, I heard from a doctor. The most recent biopsy results were 1R, and Ben had only one broken bone, the left femoral neck. (That's the part of the thigh bone that connects to the head, or "ball," located in the hip socket.)

With admirable clarity and patience, Dr. Mazen Hanna explained that "aggressive acute rehab" over the course of seven to ten days would make a tremendous and miraculous difference, even as he agreed that the broken hip was a significant variable. And he counted down what he considered the last of the clinic's checklist for Ben: dialysis was no longer needed. The trache was out. The last chest tube would be removed the next day. The orthopedic surgeon had seen Ben several times and would look at him again when the rehab folks brought him in for his next heart biopsy. Finally, while there was a slim chance that Ben would be transferred to Memorial late this week, realistically, it likely wouldn't happen until the beginning or middle of next week.

Wednesday, May 13
Full day no. 27

Hi, all—

Even as Ben has been making lots of progress (he very much wants to get out of the hospital, which means he's working hard on doing all the things they're telling him to do), I have been working since Sunday trying to converse directly with a doctor. That didn't happen until this afternoon, likely a "benefit" of his not being an SICU patient.

While there is still room for improvement, his confusion is starting to dissipate: if he gets flustered, however, it washes back over him. But in the meantime, his kidneys are working their way back to normal, his lungs are clearing up, he's graduated from a feeding tube to solid food, and they took out his trache tube this morning. They also remain pleased with how the heart is performing.

A couple more wires and tubes yet to be addressed, but the next step likely will be admission to an acute rehab facility for a length of time as yet to be defined, and then home. :-)

xoxoxo SAC

The next seven days were a blur of good days and bad days, good nights and bad nights, starts and stops. The move to rehab was scheduled, then delayed. Once. Then again. Finally, the third time proved the charm.

In the interim, medically, the last chest tube got clamped, then had to be unclamped and set back on suction because Ben couldn't tolerate the change. Blood work led to a transfusion. His trache was finally decannulated, although it would have a dressing until such time as the opening was completely healed. He experienced generalized edema, and the chest tube remained in place as the doctors waited to see additional improvement on his chest X-ray. However, nephrology officially signed off from his case, and the dialysis catheter disappeared. His blood pressure was holding steady at 110/65.

The nurses cautioned that the bedsore on his sacrum would take a long time to heal, as would the wounds in his groin area, remnants of the incisions that were made and tubes that were inserted over the course of the previous six weeks. He was getting a little bit more physical therapy each day, but that meant the pain in his left hip was severe enough for the nurses to begin administering morphine.

On the transplant front, I had a long, instructive phone conversation with Ben's transplant coordinator. She led with an apology for the fact that much of what she needed to convey was boilerplate, but it was new to me. She covered everything from care for his incision to where he should sit when in a car (in the backseat until six weeks post-transplant, i.e., June 4). No driving. No lifting of anything heavier than ten pounds. Daily checks of weight, blood pressure, temperature, and pulse. Call immediately if he develops fever, shortness of breath, fatigue, fluid retention, or general malaise. Make sure he takes his medications on time. Wear masks for six months. There would be no such thing as washing our hands too often or too much. We were to restrict visitors to people who were healthy, and all interactions, even with family, had to be socially distanced.

On the cognitive front, each day Ben checked a few more emails and sent a few more texts, slowly, slowly, slowly regaining his mental capacities. Then he begged, wheedled, and cajoled the nursing team to let him consult with Conal Ryan, our Florida Keys computer guru, to see if maybe at least the issues Ben was having with his iPad couldn't be smoothed out. When they finally agreed, I drove up to the clinic on a Thursday evening to retrieve the device, and a masked nurse came outside and extended it to me as we stood six feet apart. She looked back at the hospital and pointed to his window. It was excruciating to be so close and yet not be allowed in: I waved to the place where I thought he might be, but the panes of glass mirrored the setting sun and I couldn't see him. I cried as I found my way back to the Florida Turnpike, reached out to Conal, and handed off the iPad at a mutually agreed-upon rest area so it could be tweaked.

Late Saturday afternoon, Ben called me to FaceTime—from his *own* iPad! I answered and was stunned to see Conal standing just over Ben's right shoulder! He had talked his way into the clinic with the blessing of the charge nurse, who had capitulated because of the medical staff's concerns about Ben's ongoing confusion and potential vascular dementia; it was decided that perhaps having his hearing aids, phone, and iPad all properly synced could be therapeutic.

I was so excited by Conal's success that I woke up Sunday believing surely the hospital would let *me* visit briefly. But I was wrong.

At least I thought to ask before driving up there again. We were FaceTiming when the decision came, and I couldn't help bursting into tears. Shortly after, Ben was sobbing too, frustrated that he had to submit to the indignities of receiving hands-on assistance for every aspect of his self-care. We each needed to hang up to regain our composure. When he was able to call back a little bit later, we agreed this slog was a marathon . . . and neither of us is a marathon runner.

I spent that evening contemplating the concept of endurance. I could now see that back in March, Ben had been a growing danger to himself with each passing day and night. However, it was not until he was hospitalized, and I began to spend more time at his desk, that I finally understood how deeply compromised he was, both physically and mentally.

And now, even though he had a new miraculous, *wonderful* heart, I wasn't sure what it would take for me to believe that he and I together were either strong or wise enough to keep him safe. How would we even begin to rebuild his muscles? The transplant coordinator had suggested that walks in the park here would be good for him, and I had no doubt that in theory, they would be, but right now, because of that damn hip, he wasn't even able get out of bed or up from a chair on his own, much less walk to and from the bathroom. How long would he be on opiates? And when would he be sturdy enough for a simple (ha!) walk?

I was terrified at the dawning realization that the time when he and we needed to be toughest in this whole ordeal was likely still ahead of us.

Monday, May 18
Full day no. 32

Hi, all—

Ben's weekend was frustratingly slow and long. No major steps backward, but as the new week begins, he's only progressing in fits and starts, even as it feels like extra miles are being added to the race. The marathon is wearing on him.

While the dialysis catheter has been removed, the last chest tube is proving problematic.

It was clamped over the weekend, but today's removal was aborted. And while he has made noticeable progress in physical therapy over the past week, he is currently experiencing pain in the fractured hip, which has necessitated stronger medication. His confusion is 90 percent gone, and he can now talk briefly on the phone, but he has yet to regain the ability to concentrate well enough to engage regularly with email, texts, and phone messages.

Important good news, however, is that the doctors were pleased with the results of last Wednesday's weekly endomyocardial biopsy. In fact, he won't have to have another until at least the middle of next week.

It's mind-boggling to think Ben's had the new heart for over a month now, and each week has brought remarkable progress. We look forward to getting him home to the Keys for the summer.

xoxoxo SAC

The closer Ben came to being discharged to rehab after more than seven weeks away, the more clearly I could see that it was one thing for me to be "strong enough" to remain alone, unable to visit him in person, and quite another for me to be "strong enough" to care for him. I became obsessed with wondering how I might prepare for that. Ben's life was literally going to be in my hands, and I was terrified of messing it up royally. What well could I draw from?

That Tuesday night, I went to bed at seven thirty, half an hour before sunset, which helped "fill the well" a little.

The next morning, Ben's medical team announced that he could leave for rehab "as soon as a bed is available," and over the course of the day I fielded a flurry of calls. Midmorning, his nurse wanted to be sure I understood that his hip pain had become a major issue, and he was now taking opioids at least once a day. Ben reached out, insisting I contact some medical supply companies regarding renting a hospital bed, walker, and recliner. It was challenging to find a firm that could and would deliver quickly so far south, but finally one assured me that with two days' notice, and a substantial additional shipping and handling surcharge, they could make it happen. The social worker sent me the transfer schedule and noted that as soon as Ben left the clinic, the coordinator from rehab would be handling 99 percent of the communications regarding scheduling and what he needed medically.

Ben's nurse called again midafternoon to review the discharge instructions before he was moved to Memorial. She gave me the phone number for the hospital's pharmacy, since most of his post-transplant medications would be prescribed through there, and told me we should be watching for signs of heart failure. We were to keep a weight log; speak up regarding weight gains or losses of three or more pounds over a day or two; and note any shortness of breath, fever, redness, and puffiness anywhere, especially on the left side of the neck. We were also to keep the trache stoma covered with gauze until it healed completely, and orthopedics would be in touch two to three weeks after his discharge from rehab to discuss options regarding his hip.

As for his left leg, it was TTWB . . . I had to admit I had no idea what that was. "Toe-touch weight-bearing," the nurse said, meaning that Ben's toes could rest on the ground, but he could not put any weight on that leg. Ah, okay.

One last thing: several nurses had commented about his wild dreams and the way he talked in his sleep. For future reference, I needed to know: he was *not* to handle any reptiles—no snakes, lizards, toads, turtles, or other reptilians—for *at least* a year.

Wednesday, May 20
Full day no. 34

Good evening, all—

Late-breaking news: at 6:30 this evening, Ben arrived in his new quarters at Memorial Rehabilitation Institute, in Hollywood, Florida.

It'll likely take a day or two to figure out exactly what that means, but for now, we are rejoicing and giving thanks: He is on to the next step.

xoxoxo SAC

Our dear friends DeeDee and Terry, who'd taken a good reading of my growing fears, took me fishing on Thursday, but before we headed out, I got through to Ben's new home fairly easily and spoke with his nurse Will. After two months in bed, having medical professionals attend to his care and letting them transfer him to a gurney or wheelchair, Ben now had a full day ahead during which he'd be the primary actor doing the hard work. There were evaluations scheduled with physical and occupational therapists, a break, then a full-on occupational therapy session followed by a consult with a neuropsychologist. He'd be free again in the late afternoon but likely exhausted.

"Exhausted" was an understatement, but by the time we spoke that night, his mood had improved dramatically. He reported with enthusiasm that they'd kept him busy and paid attention to him. But what he appreciated more than anything else was that they had given him privacy in the bathroom—for the first time in eight weeks.

The rehab psychologist and I spoke on Friday. She explained that her conversation with him had been a bit challenging because he hadn't had his hearing aids in, and she noted that his hospital discharge mentioned confusion and challenges with concentration, but she assured me that the confusion already seemed to be abating somewhat and they would be working to help him rebuild his powers of concentration.

She wondered, however, what I could tell her about his mental capabilities. I explained that I knew he had a high IQ, but as for his current mental state, I was out of the loop because I hadn't seen him since March 27 and our only interactions had been via phone and FaceTime.

That said, I then mentioned one thing that had always impressed (and sometimes annoyed) me: his ability to recall conversations almost word for word.

Later in the day, I received a call from Memorial's Dr. James Salerno and Caseworker Kelly, who as a team had conferred with Ben's therapists. Based on their evaluations, Ben was found to be at a "moderate assist level," meaning that he would need help with mobility around 50 percent of the time. As for his rehab schedule, after rising, eating breakfast, and getting ready each day, he would have therapies from ten thirty to noon, be free until two thirty, then undergo additional therapies until three thirty or four.

Dr. Salerno and Kelly provided several phone numbers: for medical questions, for discharge concerns, for the charge nurse, and for the nurse assigned to him during each shift. And they said they fully expected Ben would be able to come home, riding in my low station wagon, not needing any equipment such as a hospital bed or lift chair or commode enhancement, on Wednesday, June 3, at a "modified independent supervision" level. That was *fantastic* news because it meant they expected Ben to make great and quick progress and I would not require any training. But it was *awful* news too, because it meant there was no argument to counter the facility's no-visitors pandemic protocol. I still wouldn't be allowed to visit him.

When Ben called that night, at first he was all business. He and someone named Naomi had reviewed a list of future appointments (a biopsy and heart catheterization) as well as events that would happen on the day he was discharged. I would pick him up in the late morning, and we would return to the Cleveland Clinic for a couple of appointments, first at the pharmacy, then with the pharmacist. Following that, we could return home. With those details out of the way, he exulted about how happy he was to be in a comfortable modern hospital bed.

Finally, he brought tears to my eyes when he admitted he was "hoping for a psychological step forward that hasn't come yet. It's complicated to know where I am on a scale of reality."

That at least sounded like he wanted to leave the confusion behind and find his way back to me. I fell asleep exhausted by our overwhelming two-plus months apart but grateful beyond all bounds for the joy of having a reunion date to look forward to. Thanks be to God.

Benjamin Reflects

Although I wasn't with my dad at all in person as he recovered from his transplant, the one thing that stood out to me was that he always kept his attitude and spirits up, even with everything that was going on. I could tell he was frustrated to be kept away from his hobbies (outdoor activities are hard when you need to keep your hands warm), but despite this, he always managed to keep things in perspective.

William Reflects

My dad deals with adversity much better than I do, and I was inspired by his ability to ultimately break down the realities and deal with them. He would make jokes about the situation and push on. He never felt sorry for himself in front of me in any meaningful way, and he strove to get every last drop out of the things he loved to do. I think the greatest challenge I witnessed was watching him hit new walls—realizing there were things he just couldn't do anymore. Then he would just stop, take a moment, and move on.

Friday, May 22
Full day no. 36

Hi, everyone—

Yesterday evening, at the end of his first 24 hours in rehab, Ben reported he had had a full day. The nurses, therapists, doctors, and staff had been providing "lots of care and attention," and he was looking forward to going to sleep. Late this afternoon, he reported more of the same, even as he acknowledged some frustration at the mental fogginess that keeps him from reading emails or texts or listening to phone messages. We agreed that the fog will likely continue to clear out wisp by wisp—he just needs to be patient.

But the expectation is that over the next ten days to two weeks, he will be able to complete all his activities without assistance—which is *wonderful* news because then he will be able to come home at the end of the first week of June!!!

Sometime two or three weeks later in June, the plan is to readmit him to the Cleveland Clinic to fix that fractured hip.

At the moment, however, I am so high with joy at knowing approximately when he's coming home that not being able to visit seems like a small price to pay.

Thank you and bless all of you for your love and support, especially during the eight weeks since he headed off to be admitted to the ICU.

xoxoxo SAC

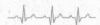

With the arrival of Memorial Day weekend, I found myself reflecting on the new and interesting turns Ben's and my conversations were taking. He could go down some rabbit holes regarding things he wanted me to deliver to rehab and how he thought his being home would have to be managed, but he also could tell that his thinking was still not clearheaded. While the mental disorder clearly frustrated him, I took tremendous comfort and found enormous relief in his recognizing it for himself. I was finally able to let myself believe it and feel it in my bones: yes, he was, at long last, on his way back to me, back to being Ben.

On Memorial Day itself, as I sat at Ben's desk to take a quick glance at the checkbook and bills, I could see that he had gone deeper into his email account than he had at any time since early April, deleting several messages and replying to others, which explained his concern during our one (very brief—he was sleepy or drugged) Sunday phone call: "There's so much I'll need to do when I get home."

"There's nothing pressing that needs your attention right now," I said. "Let's just take things one step at a time, and if we need to stand still for a bit—a moment, a day, a week—we'll do that too."

The holiday weekend also allowed me space to consider that, as sorely as I'd missed Ben's company, it would serve me well to keep in mind at all times that he had not survived this ordeal and fought to return home just to listen to me whine and blather—certainly not about any of the things I tended to obsess over or about how much I had accomplished in his absence.

There was a massive collection of cards and notes and emails to share. Perhaps when he settled in, we could go through just a few each evening and follow the conversations wherever they led. Based on his questions during several of our phone calls in the previous weeks, I knew I would do well to share upbeat stories, and to talk not so much about how generous and lovely people had been to *me* but rather about how many people had been inspired and cheered by *his* fighting spirit and resilience in the midst of this strange wrinkle in time.

There'd been so much loss. Tens of thousands from the pandemic, yes, but also Ahmaud Arbery, Breonna Taylor, George Floyd, Rayshard Brooks, Dominique "Rem'mie" Fells, Riah Milton, and too many more. So many broken hearts around the world.

One of my errands that Saturday had been to deliver a pile of Ben's "regular," easy-to-put-on-and-take-off clothes to the rehab facility along with a few other items he had requested, and it paid off on Monday morning when Ben and I had the longest back-and-forth text exchange of the previous seven weeks. The care package had included his spare hearing aids, and he remarked how beneficial it was to have working ones: he was confirming what I knew had been an issue in the hospital, but what could have been done to fix that? Now the only thing he was preoccupied with were nail clippers—they weren't allowed in rehab because of the risk of infection.

I was growing more confident as he progressed. We were a team: we could handle the upcoming battles together. It was time for me to focus on what needed to happen here at home before he returned—a few remaining move-in projects small and large, plus some serious menu planning, grocery shopping, medical equipment acquisition (three-way baby monitor, hand sanitizer, masks, gloves, a blood-pressure cuff, no-touch thermometers), and some last bits of desk work and filing in his office.

Meanwhile, the folks at rehab transported Ben to and from the clinic for his regularly scheduled biopsy. Result: 0R. Also, Ben and the physical therapist asked if I could please plan to deliver a few more items to Hollywood on Thursday. The therapist even offered Ben and me the opportunity to have a "virtual window visit."

Finally! What I had been hoping, wishing, pushing for for so long—but oh, wow, was I nervous. I arrived with incredibly detailed instructions regarding when and how to approach the front door: they had COVID systems in place for discharging patients, and I needed to not interrupt that. I waited in the parking lot until it was my time to get out of the car and walk up.

I approached the window to the left of the main entrance, just as I had been asked to do, then I heard "Sarah Cart?" from behind me. I turned to see an attendant and a patient in a wheelchair—Ben in a wheelchair . . . Ben, fifteen feet from me . . . *my* Ben, smiling. I couldn't take my eyes off him, even as the attendant, Missy, introduced herself. She was his physical therapist, and she thought it would be helpful, if I had an extra forty-five minutes, to come inside and see how his day-to-day learning routines might fit into our real life. I was stunned and thrilled and on the edge of tears. She talked me through security, and before I knew it, we were on the elevator to Ben's floor.

Thursday, May 28
Full day no. 42

Hi, all—

Today when I went to the rehab hospital to drop off some supplies, Ben's physical therapist worked some totally unexpected magic: she enabled me to visit with Ben for about 45 minutes while he did his physical therapy exercises in the facility's "home" setting. I watched him learn how to get in and out of bed and maneuver around the bathroom, and then she showed him where she'll teach him to get in and out of the car—they practice with a Mini Cooper in their "garage" setting—but that is a task for another day. He is working very hard and gets exhausted easily, but he is determined to learn what he needs to do in order to be able to function on his own.

He also had a long day yesterday—a field trip back to the clinic for one of his regular biopsies, but he was able to sit up in a wheelchair for the ride over and back, which made for a much more pleasant experience.

Our phone conversations tend to be extremely brief, but it was lovely to visit with him in person today and start to discuss how we imagine his settling in back home (at the end of next week!) will work.

It's possible that the most exciting thing for Ben was the pair of nail clippers in my pocket, which we sanitized before he borrowed them. He was hugely relieved to be able to "declaw" himself!

xoxoxo SAC

Dr. Salerno called the next day.

"Everything is still on schedule for Wednesday. You'll want some sort of home health care to come in two or three times a week—nurses to monitor his dressings, aides to help him in and out of the shower, maybe a physical therapist. The most important and immediate concern, however, is that because of ongoing cognitive dysfunction, Ben's going to require supervision whenever he's awake."

How I might choose to address that was up to me, although if I needed to do errands, for example, someone should be with him, even just "a friend with common sense." Limited executive function should come back with activities such as puzzle solving and reading, but, the doctor cautioned, "Ben will have to work his way up to the concentration levels those demand."

"I know he's anxious to get back to his desk."

"Yes, he talks about that a lot, and it will be good for his mental health, but he should not be left to his own devices with regard to your finances."

"For how long?"

"I can't tell you. It could be a week; it could be months. You'll just have to take it a day at a time."

From there, Dr. Salerno went on to talk about Ben's ongoing physical issues, most of which were gut-related, but a healthy diet and some supplements would help resolve those. He'd need to gain weight; protein would be important.

"In the meantime, do you have pen and paper? It would be a good idea to lay in a supply of certain items," and he provided a list while I scribbled as fast as I could: disposable underwear, ointment for some of his remaining wounds, a couple of handheld urinals, anti-slip socks, a waterproof mattress pad, a sturdy bedside commode, and a bed railing. They hadn't thought he'd need either of those last two items, but in consideration of that broken hip . . .

With that list in hand, I did some online shopping, then googled "cognitive dysfunction" and printed out a list of "the eight core cognitive capacities": sustained attention, response inhibition, speed of information processing, cognitive flexibility, multiple simultaneous attention, working memory, category formation, and pattern recognition. My first instinct was to think of backgammon and gin rummy—he'd always beaten me at both. We could play one or the other each night after dinner.

As June 3 approached, I was both elated and terrified, waking up in the night thinking of stuff that needed to be bought, planning menus, and making lists of foods to prepare or have on hand, mentally moving furniture to make it easier to maneuver a wheelchair or a walker around the house.

And then I'd pray: *Dear God, please please please don't let us screw up this new chapter. Help us be patient and wise as the hours and days progress.*

On Tuesday, June 2, Ben's physical therapist, Missy, called to assure me that he had the strength and mobility he needed to function at home. She wanted to be sure I understood that he would need help with such tasks as putting his pants on, and she tutored me via FaceTime in how to remove the leg rests from his wheelchair and how to fold it before putting it in the car. There was also a way to adjust the armrests, if necessary, so that he would be able to sit closer to the dinner table or his desk.

Tuesday, June 2
Homecoming Eve: Full day no. 47

Hey there, everybody—

The next chapter is about to begin: Ben officially "graduated" from rehab today and will be coming home tomorrow! :-)

I must admit I am in a bit of a panic getting ready, but it will be amazing finally to have him back in the house.

The day will be a long one. I will pick him up at rehab, along with various pieces of equipment, including a walker and a wheelchair, at 11:00 a.m. Then we are scheduled to go to the Cleveland Clinic pharmacy to collect his meds, followed by an appointment with a transplant pharmacist to review dosages and timing.

Arrival home will probably not happen until four or later, and he is already nervous about how exhausted he will be. Unfortunately, his fractured hip has proved quite painful, even as he has built up some much-needed strength and excelled at the exercises they put him through. He was quite pleased to hear from the physical therapist today that she thinks he is ready to have the hip repaired whenever the clinic says they are ready to address it. When we asked when that might be, the response was, "They will let you know."

If any of you were thinking of sending anything to honor his home-coming, please know that you are welcome to hold off for the time being, since Ben must avoid professional flower arrangements and all precut fruit, at least for the next two months (and probably longer).

But hopefully either tomorrow evening or Thursday morning as he settles in, he will be up for reading brief emails, although not necessarily responding to them yet.

Hugs and love to all—

Sarah (and Ben, soon!)

Before dawn on June 3, I noted in my journal: "Into the pinball machine we go. Plunger out. Spring taut. Chrome marble in place. Lights blinking and bells ready to chime . . . *Snap!!!* And we're off—time to set records. *Way to go, us!*"

CHAPTER 12

Tackling the Home Front

June 3, 2020—June 10, 2020

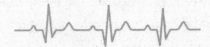

Most of the challenges presented by Ben's homecoming were overwhelming at first. But they were almost predictable—and surmountable, if broken down into smaller pieces.

Then there were the ones waiting to blindside us.

For more than two months, Ben had had the undivided attention of teams of professionals who assessed and cataloged his needs 24-7 and met each critical one instantly. Plus, in preparation for his being turned over to my care, numerous thorough and organized checklists specific to his circumstances had been prepared by doctors, nurses, therapists, nutritionists, and pharmacists.

But just as I had anticipated, from here on, accomplishing all those tasks would be up to me.

I felt responsible to Ben, the medical team, our family, and all the friends near and far who'd sustained us for so long. The full weight of these new responsibilities lay on my shoulders like that lead cape they drape over you before they take X-rays at the dentist's office.

As Wednesday dawned, I got on the road for the ninety-minute drive to rehab. It was pouring when I arrived, but I'd seen the discharge process take place with other patients just the previous week and found some comfort in that.

My phone rang. "Mrs. Cart? It's your turn."

Ben and his nurse came into view. I secured my mask and pulled up to receive my first hands-on training in helping Ben transfer from his wheelchair to the front passenger seat—we were breaking the rules by doing so one day shy of the six-week anniversary of his transplant, but Ben wanted both to be next to me and to be able to recline a little; he was very nervous about how painful the ride might prove to be and hoped that being able to adjust the seat would help. A second lesson quickly followed: how to fold and hoist his full-size chair into the back of the station wagon without stressing my back.

The nurse then handed Ben a file with all his discharge paperwork and printouts of various checklists that would help us maneuver through his continuing recovery, then returned to the rear of the car with me as we finished loading up.

"He had a dose of painkillers right before we came downstairs; hopefully they'll see him through until you get home."

"Oh, okay—good to know."

Finally, bags, boxes, and what looked like a bizarre pair of inflatable boots had all been placed in the back seat and around the edges of the folded wheelchair, and all doors had been snugged shut.

"Thank you!"

"You're welcome—and best of luck! Keep up the good work, Ben!"

We were on our way.

Masked, white-knuckled, and out of practice as a chauffeur, I barely spoke as I drove Ben back to the Cleveland Clinic for the appointments he and Naomi had scheduled at the pharmacy and with the pharmacist. Last thing I wanted to do was get us lost.

In addition to using my GPS and dealing with traffic for the first time in months, I kept running through mental checklists of my new caregiving tasks, which prompted me to ask, "Are you going to need to use a bathroom?"

"Probably, but not until we get there."

The young man at the clinic's valet parking provided additional wheelchair training, showing me how to set the brakes and adjust the footrests. We got Ben transferred, then I heaved my pocketbook and a backpack overstuffed with anything we might need—more masks, a few mini bottles of hand sanitizer, disposable gloves, a handheld urinal, clean boxers, a trash bag, baby wipes, a bottle of water, and, in case things really fell apart, a phone charger, an iPad and its charger, an extension cord, nail clippers, and a change of clothes—onto my shoulder and started to push.

Everyone entering the building had to be screened for COVID, so after properly waiting our turn, I wheeled Ben to the pharmacy, where we waited in another line before being called forward to pick up his medications.

The cheerful woman behind the window smiled behind her mask as she handed me what looked like two bagged lunches.

"Here you go, Mrs. Cart. You've got nineteen medications here, which the pharmacist will go over with you, plus a seven-day pillbox. When you need refills, give us a call. If you can't come in to pick them up, we'll overnight them to you. You should know, though, that when a prescription needs to be renewed, you'll need to call the transplant nurse first. The renewals take a bit longer because of insurance, so make those requests as soon as you can."

"Oh, wow—thank you."

From there, we negotiated the elevator and found our way to our early afternoon meeting with one of the pharmacists for a thorough discussion regarding the purpose, dosage, and timing of each of the thirty-eight-plus pills Ben would take daily. She broke down the list so that I could see what needed to go into each of the twenty-eight compartments of the new pillbox. Several drugs were to be taken more than once a day: others were morning-only and evening-only. Still others were to be taken in the late morning, midafternoon, or every other day.

"You may find that the over-the-counter meds and vitamins—acetaminophen, aspirin, zinc, and magnesium—are cheaper elsewhere. And eventually, you may want to buy an additional pillbox, but know that during these early weeks and months, some dosages will change, and some prescriptions will be discontinued. Sometimes, you'll have to go back to the filled pillboxes and adjust the meds you've already set aside."

Next, a bathroom stop in a family-friendly restroom, and finally, thanks to the valet team, we were back in the car and headed home with a good dose of Miami traffic for company.

Fortunately, Ben's adrenaline levels enabled him to tackle one of the provided checklists—the one that made accessing home health-care assistance sound easy. One after the other, he placed phone calls to arrange for a visiting nurse, physical therapist, home health aide, and occupational therapist, even as he marveled at being outside, looking at birds, cars and trucks, houses, the sky.

And I marveled too. We could do this—way to go, us.

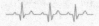

As I pulled into our garage, with its wheelchair-accessible entry into the house, Savvy appeared as she always did to greet me, full of wiggles and wags. No sooner had I opened the driver's-side door than her wiggles and wags erupted into a full-on dance. I'd brought Ben back!

The bags and boxes in the back seat needed to be carried inside, but the first order of business was to help Ben into his wheelchair. I banished Savvy to the laundry room for the moment, opened the tailgate, and unfolded the contraption. It was time for Ben to show me some of what he'd learned in rehab and teach me how best to help him. Even though we had just done this at the clinic, the valet had been there to encourage us logically from one phase to the next, and now we were on our own.

I unfolded the wheelchair and moved it as close to the passenger door as I could. Then I helped Ben find the various handles and most useful grab spots along the car's door frame. After that, I got him upright, turned around, and settled into the wheelchair, the brakes for which had been properly locked and the footrests correctly attached.

Next order of business: Savvy. The moment the laundry room door opened just far enough, she scooted through, thrilled to see and sniff to be sure that her eyes and nose had not deceived her. It was hard to tell who was more overjoyed, the pup or her master.

"Hey there, Savvy!" Ben held her face in his hands and rubbed her ears.

But before I could begin to empty the car, Ben asked, "Could you please help me get to a bathroom?"

"Do you think you can use ours?"

"No. It's gonna have to be the one where you've installed the special toilet seat and railings. And I need some pain meds."

Fortunately, the previous week's visit to rehab had helped us recognize ahead of time that rather than moving him back into the first-floor master bedroom, it would be best to set Ben up in the guest bedroom directly above—not only because he would have his own bathroom but also because the distance from the bed to the toilet was only eight feet. So I placed Ben, in his wheelchair, in the small elevator, along with his walker, and while he ascended to the second floor, Savvy and I took the stairs.

One of the many things Ben had learned was how to maneuver himself about in his new set of wheels. He treasured the smidgen of independence, but after the long day, he was happy to have my help from the elevator down the hall to "his" bedroom. Once we were at the door, however, it became obvious that while it was wide enough to accommodate the chair, jockeying the chair around two corners of the bed to the bathroom wasn't going to work.

"I'm going to have to do this with my walker." It was an obstacle course.

Notes to self: move the easy chair into the near corner; replace the shelves under the window with a folding TV table; get rid of the tripping-hazard bath mat. In the meantime, I left him to his own devices and made one quick run to grab a load out of the car, including the pharmacy packages.

When I returned, Ben took some pills, then we discussed the mechanics of the bed railing and the baby monitor with its two receivers, one in the kitchen and the other by my side of our bed downstairs, so he could ask for help if and when he needed it. I unpacked the bags I'd retrieved, and he suggested where different articles of clothing could be placed or stored so that he'd be able to find, reach, and put them on himself. He looked over the recently purchased gadget that made it possible for him to put on his own socks, pleased that it was like the one he'd used at rehab. I threw the bath mat under the bed, resituated the easy chair, and left replacing the shelves with the TV table for later.

"Do you have the energy to come back downstairs for dinner?"

"Barely, but yes. I'd like to sit in the fresh air and watch the sky change from daylight to evening and see what colors appear in the clouds."

Our angling friend Diane, anticipating our long day, had dropped off a shepherd's pie; it was sized perfectly to fit in the toaster oven so it could be warmed without overheating the kitchen. My priorities for the next few hours: feed him, manage his pain further if necessary, get his prescriptions into him, and see that he was settled into bed for the night.

I helped him wheel back into the elevator to return downstairs and made him comfortable on the back porch, where he could look over the park and watch the birds flit through the trees while I carried in more items from the car. The table there was already set, and as soon as the casserole was hot, I served it up. We'd had an incredible day, but it had been long. This was not going to be an evening for the bowl of get-well cards or gin rummy or backgammon.

I felt a bit swamped, but I was also overjoyed. To have Ben sitting there with me, so happy simply to enjoy the view and remember all the stuff on the table that we used every day but to which he'd never given a second thought. We didn't talk much, but he shared a few brief tales from his months away.

"Thank you for finding your way back to me" was about all I could say.

"We can do this, Mama Cart."

I helped him into bed, set the baby monitors so I could hear his every breath, shoved the shelves a couple of feet to the left so the TV table could nestle beside them until needed, finally finished unloading the car, and prepped a tray in the kitchen so I could carry his breakfast upstairs the instant he was ready for it the next morning.

Thursday he was up early, still on hospital time. I tried to be available as needed for his morning bathroom routine but also to stay out of the way. We charted his blood pressure, pulse, and temperature as we'd been instructed and talked about establishing some simple systems around the sink and commode to better foster his independence. Soon he was settled back on the edge of the bed with his breakfast on the TV table in front of him and the walker and his phone to the side, the baby monitor only a few feet away so he could speak up if he needed assistance.

Banana milkshake. Pills. French toast. A ramekin of butter. A small pitcher of syrup. Half a cup of coffee. A small glass of orange juice. Napkin. Silverware.

Within a couple of days, I would be able to look at a meal tray for breakfast, lunch, or dinner knowing that there was a place for everything. And when everything was not in its place, I would know instantly what was missing.

Not long after breakfast, Jo, the visiting nurse assigned to handle the initial assessment of his case, showed up, and at Ben's insistence the meeting took place in his office. Together, Jo and I decided to go through all the discharge paperwork and catalog the five wounds that needed to be addressed.

She handed me her phone and a tape measure. "This will go more quickly if you please take photos and help with measurements while I write my notes."

Because Ben had been so exhausted the night before, he'd simply stripped down to the T-shirt and special hospital-issued gauze underwear he'd worn for his homecoming; anticipating the nurse's visit, he hadn't put on much more. The three of us worked together to get him standing upright, holding on to his walker, then stripped him bare.

As I stood behind him, I bit my lip to keep from crying—he was so desperately emaciated. His discharge notes indicated that he'd lost nearly forty-five pounds. As he struggled to find his balance, his legs and arms looked barely strong enough to support him. The circumference of each thigh was scarcely more than a baseball; each bicep was smaller than a tennis ball. I resolved to move a bathroom scale into his room so we could begin tracking his weight-gaining progress.

Jo carefully examined each wound: at the base of his throat, the site of the tracheostomy; two spots on his abdomen, the remnants of drainage tubes; at the heel of one foot, skin that had been rubbed raw while he was bedridden; and at the base of his spine, a massive ten-inch-wide butterfly bedsore—one wing on each cheek with a "thorax" at the center. In order to heal, the wings needed to remain separate, and getting the bandages to stay properly in place was going to be tricky.

"Because these are all so different, they'll require different approaches. For now, let's make sure everything's clean and fresh. You'll see there are several ointments prescribed, because each does something different. And it'll be challenging to keep the area around that bedsore sterile. You may want to lay in a supply of first aid tape to reinforce the bandages at the base of the spine, since they'll be the ones most likely to come undone on their own."

Photos, dressings, and notes completed, Jo said she'd be in touch soon regarding who'd be assigned to Ben's case and suggested going online to order a few other things that would be useful in addition to the tape.

Hearing that, Ben brought up his own list. "Could you also order a cupholder and some cushions for the wheelchair? Then for the walker, another cupholder, a traveling basket, a tray, and some padded handle grips? Plus a shower chair and maybe some pajamas with elastic waistbands?"

He sounded impressively organized for someone whose doctors had been contemplating vascular dementia only a couple of weeks earlier. I smiled. "I'll see what I can do."

I saw the nurse to the door and returned to see what Ben wanted to do next.

"A nap would probably be good. And some pills. And then some lunch. Plus my hip hurts. Do you think you could get an appointment for me to get a haircut?"

After I settled him into his bed with pillows adjusted as best as possible to alleviate the pressure on his hip, I spent some time at his desk making sure all the bills and other paperwork were as up to date as possible. Jo called to say we could expect Aaron, the same young man who had been assigned to assist with Ben's course of at-home IV antibiotics three months previously, to be in touch with us soon to work out a daily schedule. She said we could count on seeing him sometime Friday.

And then the rest of the day was a blur of fetching and bringing and devising and cooking and washing and carrying and arranging . . . oh, and placing a scale in his room.

Shortly after breakfast on Friday, the physical therapist, Victor, arrived to see how he could best help us build up Ben's strength and coordination.

"This is gonna be difficult, though, because of that hip. Unless the orthopedic specialist provides me with some specific directions, I'm not sure we can accomplish much. The last thing you want me to do is make it worse."

Our being in a whole new world meant, however, that there was plenty Victor could teach us in a short time. First he confirmed that for now the only way Ben could get in and out of the house was via the ramp in the garage, despite our hopes that he'd be able to manage the two steps to the front door. That was frustrating, but we were glad to have a professional make the assessment.

Then he gave us various hands-on transfer lessons, showing me how to use a gait belt to help bear some of Ben's weight and offering invaluable advice about how to get Ben in and out of the walk-in shower and onto the shower chair once it arrived. Especially helpful was Victor's observation that, because the broken hip was Ben's left, he would have a tough time using the shower in "his" bathroom, with its door that opened out and to the right.

"Does the shower in that bathroom closer to the office have a door that opens the other way, by any chance?" It did, and while we didn't plan to try it on our own, we felt better prepared for the eventual arrival of the home health aide.

Victor returned Saturday, and we practiced and perfected the transfer scenarios he had laid out the day before, but with no further direction from the doctors, we finally agreed with Victor's judgment that physical therapy was not appropriate for the time being, which meant we needed to bid him farewell.

"Good luck to you; maybe I'll be back once the hip's been fixed."

"Thanks, Victor. And thank you for being so frank."

As for Aaron, the nurse assigned to take on the day-to-day responsibilities of cleaning and evaluating Ben's wounds and changing his dressings, we didn't hear from him until Friday afternoon. He was happy to say hello, and "Congratulations on the new heart!" And "How frustrating about the broken hip!" But, well, his schedule was tight—there was no way he could get to all his clients in Miami *and* get down to the Keys to help Ben before the end of business, but he'd read Jo's assessment, and he assured me all five dressings would be okay for another day. We'd see him midday Saturday.

While I'd been relieved that there would be professional assistance from someone who knew how to find our home and whom we had already met, I had worried about just this scenario. During that previous go-round, months earlier, after Aaron gave me an initial lesson in IV administration, he never quite grasped that he needed to show up twice a week, and most of our interactions had consisted of his "supervising" my work via telephone. That had been at the very beginning of COVID, however, when the country had suddenly shut down and before any protocols had been set. Now that Ben was recovering from a heart transplant, I'd hoped Aaron would step up and arrive every day as scheduled.

But when Saturday evening arrived with no word, I texted him to ask, "What's up?"

"Sorry—can't get there today, either."

"So you're sending someone else instead?" No response.

In the meantime, we'd finally heard from the home health aide. She'd begged off because she didn't want to come until after Aaron's visit. She mentioned that if we could get Aaron to provide a schedule, she would dovetail her subsequent visits so she could help Ben get his showers right before Aaron's arrivals. That way Aaron could reapply the various medications and all five dressings.

Ben had now been in my care for eighty hours; I was mastering keeping him fed and medicated and charting his blood pressure, temperature, and weight. (He hadn't gained an ounce, and had in fact probably lost a few.) But he hadn't had a shower in three days or clean bandages in two. I felt vastly underqualified to resolve either situation.

By 8:30 p.m., I'd lost it and soon hit Send on a flaming text:

Aaron, as you know, Ben got a heart transplant. He's on massive doses of immunosuppressants that put him at grave risk of infection. He has numerous wounds, including a bedsore that's seeping. All the dressings are to be changed daily, but none has been changed since Thursday morning. He needs a professional to look each wound over, clean it, rebandage it, and assess his progress. I am not qualified to do that. He has a painful broken hip that the doctors won't address until the bedsore is under control, and the home health aide can't schedule a time to come over and help him shower until she knows *you'll* arrive shortly after her regular visits, so he has not had a shower since leaving rehab on Wednesday. If you cannot get here *tonight*, either you or I need to get First Agency Healthcare to send someone else. *Now.*

My chest was tight, my stomach had turned to stone, and my head throbbed. Our local medical center was a wonderful resource, but it was only open during the day, and it wasn't an urgent-care facility. What was I going to do?

In the end, Aaron rearranged some things and managed to arrive at 10:00 p.m. Ben went to bed that night with clean bandages. Heading out the door, Aaron avoided looking me in the eye. "I'll call my supervisor tomorrow to suggest that the agency assign someone else as soon as the new work week begins."

Sunday came and went without a word.

Monday morning, Ben and I were up early. There wasn't time to address the Aaron issue because we were preparing for a "quick" 150-minute round-trip to the hospital for a COVID test in anticipation of a biopsy later in the week. Ben needed to eat his breakfast and take enough pain meds to make the road trip bearable, and I was working on filling the backpack that would become our go bag for such trips through the weeks ahead. Part of the push was that we needed to be back by 10:30 a.m. for Ben's "post-hospital check-in" with Carlos. And as soon as we got home from that, I'd give Ben his lunch and help him go down for a nap. Then I would finally reach out to First Agency Healthcare (FAH) to hammer out better home-care options. But before we'd even pulled out of the garage, an incoming text pinged on Ben's phone.

Aaron: "I'll be there at 1:30 p.m. today."

And he was, except that by then the changing of Ben's bandages was a moot point; Carlos's team had already handled it.

Tuesday, nothing. No texts. No house call.

Wednesday morning, Ben's phone pinged as he was eating breakfast. "Hi, Ben. Aaron here. Can't get there today. Maybe tomorrow."

I was furious—yet another day without the support we needed, and the next day was slated to be another early and, this time, full day at the hospital, beginning with a 6:00 a.m. catheterization and concluding nearly eight hours later. I was already obsessing about what time we'd need to be up and out of the house.

As Ben answered Aaron's text, I dialed FAH on my phone. A woman answered almost immediately, but the conversation quickly devolved.

From her position of pseudo authority, she suggested that no matter what the prescribing doctor said, Ben's wounds didn't *really* need daily care, and, "well, since you're planning to be at the clinic tomorrow for a full day anyway, maybe if you feel so strongly that a nurse should dress his wounds, perhaps you should have a nurse there change his bandages for you."

She might more accurately have declared that FAH's priority had nothing to do with the prescribed care and everything to do with getting the insurance money.

I was apoplectic.

"Arranging to change those bandages is FAH's job, *not* the hospital's. Please figure out how you're going to make that happen and let me know ASAP."

"Well, maybe we can find someone to get out there today, but I can't promise anything."

After hanging up, I tried to reach the social worker at rehab but could only leave a message.

Fury evolved to panic. Ben had been home for one week, and the systems we'd been told (assured, *promised*) would fall into place were failing us. How were we going to get by?

I was managing to feed him three high-calorie meals and several snacks each day. I was helping him get to and from the bathroom (cleaning up accidents as necessary), ensuring he was taking the correct doses of his medications on time, trying as best I could to help him find the least uncomfortable ways to accommodate his hip, answering his phone and taking messages for him when he napped, and sneaking at least twenty minutes at his desk after he went to bed to ensure that all was in order with the bills and his emails, plus taking the stairs three at a time whenever he whispered to the baby monitor, "Are you there? I need some help."

I was baffled by the unreliability of the prescribed support services. Was it because of the pandemic? Or because we lived out of the way, in the Keys? I couldn't get answers. I had no idea where to turn to get results. I'd already made inquiries about private-duty nurses only to be told, "Not now. COVID means everyone's booked solid. There's no one around."

I was afraid that daily nursing care existed only in our imaginations.

Ben hadn't had a shower in more than a week, but it felt risky and stupid to blend his instability with my bad back, some glass, some tile, and a lot of water and shampoo and soap. The counterweight to that, though, was that any one of his wounds could develop into an issue that might delay resolution of the hip situation.

Complicating matters was my finally experiencing in person what Dr. Salerno had warned me about: despite his impressive list-drafting abilities, displayed that first morning home, and despite my so wanting those to be a sign, Ben wasn't "all there" mentally. The glitches were subtle but real.

Already he had decided that we should lease our cabin up North for much of the summer and had nearly made promises we couldn't keep—including that surely we'd be up there for two or three months in the fall. He was exceedingly fretful about cash flow, and despite having managed the books for the previous two months, I remained naive as to exactly why that was. True, our old house just around the corner had yet to sell, but the real estate agents were showing it regularly and felt sure an offer would be forthcoming. Perhaps Ben's angst was a manifestation of residual paranoia from his hospital nightmares about our being embezzled. Plus, the day before, on Tuesday, he'd gotten out ahead of his physical capabilities, reaching too far to open a file cabinet drawer, and fell in his office.

I'd been coming up the stairs at the time and heard the thump. I raced to his office. "Ben!"

"I'm fine! I'm fine!"

"What were you doing?!"

"Sorry—I was just trying to remember what was in that drawer and thought I'd check it out."

"Why?! Wait—forget I asked. Does anything hurt? I won't dare try to pick you up, or we'll both end up back in the hospital."

Fortunately, he really did appear to be okay, if a bit bemused to find himself sprawled on the floor, but for me it was terrifying proof that, for the moment at least, he remained a danger to himself. Thankfully, when I called the local security guard and Alfredo, they arrived within minutes, and Ben thought to suggest the gait belt as a means of levering him off the floor and setting him upright again; for one brief instant, I was grateful he weighed so little.

And there were the unpredictable mood swings, from that calm bemusement after his fall to a snippy grouch I hardly recognized and then back to the guy I'd fallen in love with more than four decades ago.

That same night, when I suggested that a different route to the lavatory than the one he was considering would give him a straighter, easier shot and would make maneuvering the wheelchair more manageable, he blasted me.

"*Well* then, whatever *YOU* say must be right!"

He had never, ever spoken to me, or anyone, with such snark.

Stung, exhausted, and reeling at how things seemed to be spinning out of control, I snapped.

"God*damn* it! This *isn't* about me. It's *all* about you. *Everything* I have done since you got home has been for *you*. *Your* meals. *Your* appointments. Racing upstairs whenever the baby monitor squawks. Indulging your choice to spend *hours* in your office obsessing over the summer schedule and fixating on how you're going to get back to Pennsylvania by October so you can climb into a deer stand. You're counting the days till then because it's all about *you*. If you'd take ten seconds to look at last week on that same calendar you're so hyperfocused on, you might have noticed I had a birthday!"

I burst into tears.

He opened his eyes wide and looked at me, shocked. "Oh! Oh, I am so sorry. I'm sorry." And then his eyes were damp. "All I can give you is a hug."

It was awkward letting him do so as he sat in the chair, and I ended up sobbing on his chest . . . listening to his heart beat.

In my head, I knew it was the most amazing, miraculous birthday present ever, and I was grateful that we'd been given this astounding opportunity, but the daily responsibilities were beyond overwhelming.

CHAPTER 13

The Fog of War

June 10, 2020—June 12, 2020

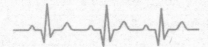

After that disastrous Wednesday morning interaction with the woman at FAH, I needed to get out of the house. Ben was ready for a nap, and he had his phone, so I told him to call me if he needed me. Then I escaped for a ten-minute walk, hoping to bring my blood pressure and heart rate back within striking distance of normal and trying to imagine how we could proceed.

When I got back into the house, the message light on the landline's answering machine was flashing.

"Hi. My name is Gretel. I'm an LVAD RN [cardiac nurse] with First Agency Healthcare and will be there between four thirty and five this afternoon."

I raced upstairs to tell Ben. He was awake and already knew because she'd also texted and called his cell phone, but the message he'd taken away from the call was different.

"She told me we should call FAH and tell them to send the orders to Charles at Twofold Health Agency, and she gave me Charles's number. Apparently she freelances for both, and she says Twofold is better."

Had we heard of Twofold before? It sounded vaguely familiar. Wasn't that the agency that had overseen the IV antibiotics three months ago? So Aaron freelanced too?

I called FAH to ask that they please forward the orders to Twofold. The request was not well received; they weren't going to be forwarding any orders to anyone.

"You're going to have to contact the prescribing doctor." I called Charles at Twofold.

"You need to call either your insurance company, the rehab doctor or social worker, or maybe all three."

The runaround was still in full swing when Gretel showed up.

Her response when I said the switch wasn't going well was to dismiss it. "Don't worry about it. I'm here now. I can fix it. You're in good hands; you just need to breathe."

I almost believed her.

First, she instructed me to pay no attention to the brace on her right wrist. "I'm left-handed and the fingers on my right hand still work, so it's no big deal, but there's a funny story behind it—I had a client who'd had a forklift drive over his foot and the doctors wanted to amputate, but I told them that wasn't acceptable and refused to let the patient give up hope. It took a long time, but I saved it, and then on the very last visit, I tripped getting into my own car in his driveway and *whoops!* Broke my wrist! Go figure! But a small price to pay to have been able to save his foot. By the way, do you mind if I use your restroom?"

"No, of course not. Please go ahead." I showed her to the lavatory just inside the front door.

This had to be the angel we'd been waiting for.

She explained that she hadn't wanted to use a restroom at the gas station because of COVID. She added, "I don't want to put my gloves on until we're dealing with Ben's dressings, especially since I need an extra large one to fit over the brace and I don't have a 'huge' (get it?!) supply of those, but don't worry, I won't touch the doorknob."

She settled into the lav without closing the door. It felt awkward, but . . . she was here, and she was COVID-conscious. These were blessings. Except then the landline rang, so I had to walk directly by the open door.

It was the social worker calling to ask how things had settled out. I reported that FAH appeared to have gotten its act together, because the fill-in nurse had arrived.

"So you're okay with First Agency Healthcare continuing?"

"Well, yeah, I think so. They've finally sent a replacement nurse. So yes."

When Gretel emerged from the lav, she indicated she was ready to meet Ben. We headed to his office, and after brief introductions and a discussion of the five dressings that needed to be changed, she set to work, recruiting me as an extra set of hands and asking me to take baseline photos with her phone, just as Jo had had me do seven days before.

The tracheostomy site was nearly healed, but Gretel wanted a new dressing on that site. What materials did we have on hand? I had laid out everything Jo had suggested but wondered, Wasn't the agency supposed to provide this stuff? Or were folks just supposed to know what to buy? And how did most people afford this or manage all the insurance paperwork?

The groin site where they'd gone in for the catheterizations was also nearly healed, but Gretel's assessment was that, no, that would need a different kind of dressing.

The sores on his feet?

"Oh, those look awful," she declared, and she instructed me that Ben needed to be able to rest at night with his feet elevated on pillows in such a way that his heels couldn't rub against anything. I wasn't sure she understood that with his broken hip, once he'd managed to find the least painful position to curl up and sleep in, there was no way I was going to say, "Oh, but your heels need to be elevated and hanging over the edge of these pillows so you don't rub them raw."

Finally, she was ready to address the sacral wound at the base of his spine. We helped Ben stand up, using his walker for support, and stripped him from the waist down.

"Oh, my goodness, you poor man! Has anyone been taking care of this?!?" Obviously, the FAH staff hadn't let on how unreliable their support had been so far.

Gretel had plenty to say. She went on at length about the buddy whom she'd helped for free . . . her medical training . . . her friend the state representative . . . the client who lived in the same neighborhood as the hospital, so we could stop there on the way home tomorrow without her having to come all the way out to the Keys—wait, what?—and the other friend who had vacant office space on US 1 who'd surely let us meet there for just an hour . . . Oh, dear.

And yet she treated each wound, enlisting me as her accomplice at every step, having me unwrap saline syringes, provide squares of gauze and Q-tips daubed with a special "butt cream," and help tape the edges of each bandage to ensure it would stay.

"Don't worry; we've got this, Ben. I'm here for you now, and I'll see you through, whatever it takes."

As the exercise ended, she promised, "I'll text you tonight to let you know what kind of dressings to buy—they make special sacral ones."

At last Ben was settled back into his wheelchair, and I walked her through the house, headed for her car.

"Do you mind if I wash my hands one more time before I leave? Let's go in the kitchen so you can write down a to-do list at the same time."

As she managed to scrub despite her braced wrist, I took notes as directed.

"The moment you arrive at the hospital tomorrow, you need to ask for a charge nurse. You want a wound care specialist to see him at some point during the day before you leave there. And his diet is critical"—as if the nutritionists at both the hospital and rehab hadn't alerted me to this and as if I hadn't devoted days to drafting lists of ingredients and menus and groceries, both before he'd come home and since.

"Who's his transplant coordinator?"

I mentioned one of the three we'd been working with.

"Oh, really? Wow. I know her—we trained together. I wondered where she ended up." That was odd. My recollection was that this coordinator had moved to Florida from Ohio only a year earlier, whereas Gretel had been born, raised, and educated in Florida, or so she told me.

"You know, there are lots of great orthopedic surgeons in Miami. You don't have to go back to the clinic to get his hip fixed. You should be getting a second opinion. He needs that surgery *now*."

I was so conflicted. I'd wanted so badly for this woman to be the answer to my prayers, to resolve my issues and fears about how home health care was going, but the past hour (or had it been two by now?) had been exhausting.

"I love the colors you've decorated with. Are you German, by any chance? I'm German—that explains our similar tastes."

This was becoming grossly uncomfortable.

"Here's another thing: absolutely *no* spinach or dark green vegetables. They don't digest well. *No* tomatoes. *Nothing* that might give him gas. *No* sugars . . ."

I heard whispers deep in my head: the rehab doctor telling me that spinach and kale and Swiss chard were all high in magnesium, and getting those into his diet was going to be critically beneficial for his gut. The nutritionist recommending the protein drinks, even though they were loaded with sugar, because at this point the calories were more important. Ben needed to heal *and* gain weight.

Ugh. Gretel was still talking. "You're going to need a special ice pack for him. Coldest is the best brand. Look it up—it's the kind all the professional athletes use."

My head went to his Raynaud's and his issues with even minor changes in temperature.

As for which agency would be overseeing this assignment, we didn't need to worry; she'd take care of that. She just needed a copy of the front and back of Ben's insurance card. I gave her the one that was pinned to the kitchen bulletin board.

At last, we were headed out the front door, but then she turned to me and stiffened. "You know, it's just amazing that he got a heart. I've got friends who've been on the list for years, and he was on the list for what? When did you say he was listed—early April? And surgery was a few days after Easter? Not even two weeks?"

She shook her head in disbelief. "Wow."

Now she was finally at her car door, but she still wasn't leaving. She looked at me over the roof of her car.

"You look awfully tired. How's your sleep? Have you tried meditation? It would do you good. Plus, I can tell you're too nice. *You* are *his* advocate, the only one he's got. You need to yell and get people's attention. Be sure to call me as soon as you're back on the road from the hospital tomorrow so I can let you know where we should meet for his dressing changes."

She climbed in and drove away.

I didn't know whether to feel relieved or weirded out. Ben had clean dressings, but at what cost?

When I went back to check on him in his office, he was the most relaxed I'd see him in days and visibly more comfortable. It had been a stressful week: maybe I was just being overly paranoid. Gretel had talked far more than felt appropriate, but she *was* a cardiac nurse and obviously incredibly dedicated. All things considered, we were far ahead of where we'd been before her visit.

Ben was in such good humor that I suggested maybe, even if we didn't feel confident about getting him in and out of the shower, I could wash his hair. All he'd need to do was stand at the kitchen sink for a few minutes while I went after him with the sprayer. We were both soaked by the end, but there'd been some laughs, and he looked fresh in anticipation of the next day's road trip to and from the clinic.

By the time we were seated at the dinner table, we were reflecting on how lucky we were that, after five days of what had felt like fruitless efforts to get home nursing care in place, perhaps things were finally on track. And tomorrow was going to be hectic—each of us had lists of what we'd need for the car and for the long day at the hospital: the walker, the wheelchair, the footrests for the wheelchair, a small cooler with some water, the meds (in a baggie) Ben would be allowed to take before the procedure, lunch, snacks, and the other meds he was supposed to take midmorning and midafternoon (in a second baggie), plus all his meds in their original containers *and* the chart of his daily morning weight, blood pressure, temperature, and pulse, since those were supposed to be shown to the doctors at every appointment.

When asked, Ben admitted he thought he'd need to be awakened by 3:30 a.m. in order to be ready to depart at four thirty, so we agreed that we had to get to bed by nine or nine thirty at the latest.

But then a text came in from Gretel, and then another, and another, followed by a 9:00 p.m. phone call that began with, "Don't mind me. I'm just in the drive-through line at my pharmacy picking up some pain meds for my wrist—I'll tell you what: I could have a second career as a weather forecaster. I was thinking as I sat here waiting, you may want to get silver-infused sacral bandages—wait a sec . . ."

Then to someone else, "Yes, my birthdate is August 24, 1964 . . . that's right, eight twenty-four sixty-four . . . okay, thanks!"

Then she was talking to me again, dictating the address of her friend's vacant office on US 1 and instructions for how to reach her when we were finally headed back to the Keys from Weston the following afternoon so we could meet at the office en route, and lastly offering to forward links to products on Amazon . . .

I struggled to fall asleep, agonizing over the insanity of all Gretel had said and promised.

Were we really this desperate? And if not, at what point were we supposed to say, "No, thank you. You need to leave"? And if we did so, what other options did we have?

Ben Reflects

During this time, I wasn't sure if I was ever going to get better, so I spent a lot of time focusing on making sure Sarah's life was going to be right if I died. In fact, I was much more worried about her than I was about myself.

In taking care of me, she was totally out of her element. I was the scientist in the family, and she was the English major. It was always my job to deal with blood. That's just not what she did. So for her to face major medical explanations and decisions was very challenging. Not to mention the difficulties with my home care. Sure, we got help, but it wasn't always competent, nor was it full-time. So Sarah was forced to deal with my IVs and tend to my bedsores and work on my feet—all these incredibly unfamiliar and distasteful things. Talk about being out of your comfort zone!

In a sense, she had to swallow everything about herself to take care of me. Throughout it all, she was deeply devoted to not losing me, whether for my own sake or for herself. I'm sure it was both.

It felt like only a moment later when the alarm went off.

We bid a nervous Savvy farewell and headed off in Thursday's pre-dawn dark. Not knowing whether I'd be permitted in the hospital, I'd prepared for the possibility of a long hot day in the parking lot, with files and paperwork that could be addressed on my laptop as I sat in the wayback of my station wagon with the tailgate open. As it turned out, so long as Ben was in the wheelchair, I would be allowed—and sometimes expected—to push him from appointment to appointment, starting at the admitting department.

I asked about talking with a charge nurse and seeing a wound care specialist, but at the clinic, that meant a plastic surgeon, and we'd need a physician's referral for an appointment with that department. The charge nurse wasn't a possibility. At every opportunity—the blood lab, the cath lab, X-ray, cardiology—we mentioned the bedsores. Finally, Dr. Manrique, the orthopedic surgeon, asked to see the big one, especially since it was the highest hurdle we'd need to clear before scheduling the operation to fix his hip.

"Wow. Yes, that is a serious wound."

He made clear that the biggest risk with hip replacement is infection, and bacteria love metal, and while he could see how much pain Ben was in and how anxious we were to get on his surgical calendar, there wasn't really a choice but to wait until all Ben's wounds were healed before performing a total hip arthroplasty. It might take a month; three weeks if we were lucky. In the meantime, recognizing that Ben had already been on opioids since mid-May and was therefore technically "addicted," Dr. Manrique gave us a referral for pain management.

"The more we do now to minimize your use of those medications, the more effective they'll be when you really need them, which will be in the days right after the hip is repaired." He immediately asked his assistant to schedule a FaceTime telehealth session with the pain management doctor as early as possible the next morning.

She returned less than a minute later. "Will 11:00 a.m. work?"

"Yes, thank you."

Dr. Manrique also shared some of the specifics about the operation and mentioned that we might want to consider a Girdlestone procedure, which would remove the broken bone and shorten the length of Ben's leg but relieve some of his pain. It would be a stopgap measure to be followed up with a proper replacement later, but that decision could wait. When Ben finally headed in for surgery, some meds might have to be adjusted or reduced in the days before to "optimize" him. Anesthesia would be a spinal, and the incision would be at the front of the hip. Typical recovery is two to six weeks. Ben would be up and walking the same day, but he'd spend at least one night in the hospital. It was a ton of information to process, but we were grateful for Dr. Manrique's attention to detail and his obvious concern and desire to help move Ben's recovery along as quickly as possible.

"Let's stay in close touch. Take down my cell phone number and send me photos every few days of the progress with the wounds, especially that bedsore. You say you have home health coming in daily to clean it and change the bandages?"

"Why, yes, um, finally. Yes. Yes, we do."

"Then keep doing what you're doing. Send those photos, and we'll talk again in two weeks."

It had been an exhausting eight hours of appointments and procedures and waiting rooms and elevators and family restrooms and long corridors and masks and sanitizer and temperature checks, but now it was time to head home and figure out exactly where and how today's nursing visit was going to work. The young man at valet parking helped me fold Ben and his walker and his wheelchair back into the car, and I got us onto the highway while Ben used his cell phone to call Gretel.

Typically, I cannot hear the other person on Ben's calls because they're routed through his hearing aids, but this time, even over the sound of the trucks and other traffic on the highway, within moments it was clear that Gretel had asked a question, didn't like the answer, and now was raging. Ben, who used to lose his temper so rarely, was furious.

"*No*, we did *not* see a wound care specialist. We got through blood work and a catheterization and X-rays and a meeting with the orthopedic surgeon, and I'm exhausted and need to get home. So no, we're not meeting you at some vacant office next to US 1. You're gonna need to follow agency protocol and come to the house."

He hung up, but she texted back repeatedly and called his cell and mine to leave messages.

"You're right. Of course you're exhausted. You're the one who got the transplant . . ." Next voice mail: "This is what Sarah should have done on your behalf . . ."

A few voice mails after that: "I'm sorry, Ben, but without new orders, my hands are tied. I'm not going to be able to meet you this afternoon."

That drove Ben to call her back.

"So you won't be coming to the house? Or are you saying some other nurse will be coming?"

"Sorry, Ben. Can't talk right now. I'm on the road; gotta go." Click.

We arrived home to find two messages on the landline's answering machine. "Good afternoon. I'm calling from First Agency Healthcare to let you know that no authorized nursing visits remain." No name, no time, no callback number.

Second message: "Hello, this is Synchronized Basics, Inc. We're calling on behalf of Ben Cart's insurance company to verify that home nursing services have been provided to him by First Agency Healthcare. Please ring us back."

I made dozens of phone calls Thursday evening and Friday—to the transplant coordinator, the social worker at the hospital, the social worker at rehab, First Agency Healthcare, Twofold, and Synchronized Basics, the insurance company's middleman (an 866 number, so I was repeatedly talking with a new agent, but each one promised to "escalate" Ben's case).

The only "break" was Friday morning's FaceTime telehealth appointment with Dr. Giraldo about pain management.

He began by explaining, "If you've been taking oxycodone for more than two weeks, you are already dependent. Moving forward, track your pain on a scale of 1 to 10. When it's less than 5, take Tylenol. If it's greater than 6, take the oxy."

He then cautioned, "Whatever combination you take, do not exceed four pills a day. And don't take ibuprofen. One of its side effects is that it compromises bone's ability to heal."

Before signing off, he advised, "And although I know you won't want to hear this, you need to move as much as you can; medicate before moving. Let's talk again in a week to review how all this works for you and renew your oxycodone scrip if necessary."

Still exhausted by the previous day's exertions, and dispirited by these new marching orders, Ben just wanted to nap. We made every effort to get him as comfortable as possible, then I returned to working the phones to resolve the home health-care issues, becoming more desperate with each call.

Not wanting to wake Ben, I took to screaming into a pillow every time I hung up, and by midafternoon my vocal cords felt like I'd massaged them with sandpaper. I was making some sort of strange progress, however, because several agents from Synchronized Basics called back as Friday afternoon turned to evening.

Finally, yet another Synchronized Basics rep reached out, but this one used the word "expired" for the first time regarding the rehab hospital's orders for home nursing.

I'm sorry—what??

Despite its being after hours, I called rehab to ask that the orders be renewed. Mere minutes later, even though he wasn't on call that weekend, Dr. Salerno phoned me directly.

He was *livid*.

"I *never* issue orders that are less than four weeks in duration. There is *no way* they have expired." He gave me a long pep talk regarding patients' rights and the agency's potential exposure for liability if it did not follow through, especially in the state of Florida.

"You have rights. That agency is liable if it fails to provide what it was contracted to provide."

While I felt (somewhat) vindicated after all the fruitless phone calls of the past forty-eight-plus hours, Ben had once again gone for more than twenty-four hours without getting his dressings changed. It had been a long day at the end of a long week. I determined that our only option was to visit Carlos's nurses the next morning, taking along all the prescribed ointments as well as the silver-infused sacral bandages Gretel recommended, which had just arrived. And since we appeared truly to be on our own, we were going to have to brave Ben's taking a shower.

But for now: bed and a beautifully timed caring email from a faraway friend. Although it couldn't fix the mess we were in, it raised my spirits.

Friday, June 12

Dear Sarah:

As different people respond to your updates and as we think about where we would have been if the world hadn't imploded—including but not limited to a husband getting a heart transplant—I continue to think about you.

Hopefully Ben continues to make progress and the fog continues to lift on his brain.

Hopefully your men and their families are all healthy and safe. Hopefully all the loved ones you take such good care of can now take care of themselves and you might—maybe?—have a minute to take care of you.

I wish for you a weekend of love, laughter, and knowledge that you have done mighty work on this planet for a long time, especially in the past few months.

Thinking of you with a smile and a song,

Betsy

CHAPTER 14

Battle Stations

June 13, 2020—June 23, 2020

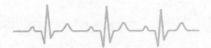

After breakfast Saturday morning, we headed to see Carlos at our community's medical center, where Ben was now a local hero of sorts. All the staff members there had been aware of his declining health over the previous three years, and now found inspiration in his having received a heart transplant in the midst of the ongoing pandemic. If he had a broken hip and a bedsore, well, so be it: we simply needed to move forward one battle at a time, and they let us know with their masked smiles and congratulations that they would be there to help us as best they could.

Apologizing for not being able do anything to ease the home health-care situation, Carlos gave all Ben's wounds a good looking over and had his nurse, Dani, apply all new dressings as well as schedule another appointment to do more of the same come Monday. Though waiting another forty-eight hours to get them changed again wouldn't be ideal, at least we could plan on that if nothing else fell into place, and if the past ten days were any indication, that felt like a good bet.

We returned home, and I set Ben up on the porch to enjoy his lunch.

As he was finishing, he took a call on his cell. It was a young woman (he hadn't caught her name), working with some government department (he hadn't caught that, either), who needed to talk with him in person this afternoon about some case that had been opened; she was the one on call this weekend in Miami. She'd be at our place by three thirty or so.

How curious. Our first thought was *Oh, wow! Someone's looking out for us!* With that in mind, Ben had time for a nap, and then we set him up in his office.

At three twenty-five, I opened the front door to a lovely soft-spoken African American woman.

"Mrs. Cart? I'm Sasha. I'm a caseworker with the Florida Department of Children and Families. I'm here regarding a complaint filed about elder abuse and neglect. By law, that requires an on-site interview within twenty-four hours. I'm here to speak with your husband."

When she asked Ben if it would be okay if she spoke with him alone, he laughed and said, "You could try, but I'll miss a lot of what you're saying, especially since I can't read lips when you're wearing a mask. If you don't mind, I'd like Sarah to stay—she's my 'translator.'"

For an hour, Sasha asked Ben all kinds of questions, some of which he caught and many of which he missed because Sasha was so soft-spoken. I restated those for him, but anytime I began to coax him with the start of an answer, because that might help him better understand the question, Sasha would caution me.

"No—I need *his* reply." Not saying, but strongly implying, "No coaching."

Meanwhile, Ben was reveling in this: an engaging young person asking him to share the story of his transplant and what it was like to return home after our having been apart for nearly ten weeks; how much his hip hurt and how frustrated he was to have a souvenir bedsore delaying getting the hip replaced; how thrilled he was to be able to sleep—or at least rest, depending on the pain—through the night in a dark room and be done with hospital food; how many pills he had to take a day and how we were managing his pain medications. And so much more.

As the interview drew to a close, Sasha indicated that she had a few pieces of paperwork he needed to sign, allowing her department to look over our bank accounts and access his health records.

Once the ink had dried, I escorted Sasha back to her car, giving her a tour on the way—of Ben's room and bathroom and the elevator and the handicap ramp in the garage and the kitchen and the contents of the fridge (overflowing with protein drinks) and the ice cream in the freezer and the bananas for his milkshakes to boost his potassium and the food cupboard and the posted lists of menu ideas and the tray already set up to be filled with his dinner and the box of his medications and his filled pillboxes and what had become many go bags stuffed with all the paraphernalia that we needed to take with us whenever he had an appointment at the clinic . . .

As we stepped out the front door, I dared ask, "You mentioned that this interview was required because a complaint has been filed."

"That's correct."

"Was it anonymous?"

"No, but I am not at liberty to identify the source."

"And your job is to substantiate it?"

"Yes, one way or the other, true or false. Filing a false complaint is a felony or misdemeanor. Someone from our office will be in touch within forty-eight hours."

When I walked back into Ben's office, he looked befuddled. He'd been looking through the quarter-inch-thick pile of paperwork she'd left with him and rereading the copies of everything she'd had him sign.

"According to this, her job is to protect 'vulnerable adults from further abuse, neglect, exploitation, or self-neglect.' Why was she here? What do you think all that was about?"

"I think by the state's definition, you are a vulnerable adult, and the wrong answer to one or two of her questions could result in either you or me being removed from our home."

"That can't happen—can it?"

"I don't know."

We didn't talk much through dinner except to wonder, "Who, do you think?"

"Gretel? She certainly had a lot to say and a lot of schemes. She may have thought we were going to report her, so she decided to strike first. And she was awfully suspicious of your getting a transplant so 'easily.' The fact that you were dying didn't impress her."

"Or Dr. Salerno? You said he was awfully angry."

"Maybe. Who knows what kind of history he's had with FAH? I suppose if he thought it would get them to fulfill their obligation he might have."

"But all of this is just speculation, we really don't know."

While over the past week we had taken up alternating between backgammon one night and gin rummy the next, neither of us was up for games this evening.

After I'd cleared the dishes and returned to the table with a bowl of banana pudding and some Nilla wafers for Ben's dessert, he asked, "Do you think we need a lawyer?"

"I was wondering about that too. Yeah, I'm afraid I think maybe we do."

At 8:00 p.m., I texted a brief outline of the circumstances to a judge we'd known socially for a few years, with apologies for bothering him on a weekend. Despite its being a Saturday night, he responded within half an hour to advise us that what we needed was a malpractice lawyer who specialized in family law. He gave us a name and a phone number and advised, "Call him tonight."

By 9:00 p.m., we'd left a message on that lawyer's answering machine.

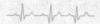

The next day was the quietest one we'd had since Ben's discharge from rehab. The only professional input was a call from Synchronized Basics to report that Ben's case had been passed along to another home health-care agency, Redux. We could expect to hear from the people there first thing Monday.

"That's good news, thank you. But just in case they're too swamped to reach out to us, would you please give me their phone number?" I was learning.

Monday. A new week. A new beginning. A brief but calming return call from the malpractice lawyer. And another visit to Carlos and his team for new bandages. But when by 4:00 p.m. there'd been no word from Redux, I called.

"Any chance you can tell me what's up?"

"We can't initiate care until we've received doctors' orders." I called Carlos's office and Synchronized Basics.

Each reported, "Orders were sent this morning." I called Redux again.

"Can you give us your insurance company's contact information? We'll call you back shortly."

As Tuesday dawned, Ben was two months post-transplant, and disappointingly, all remained quiet on the home-health-agencies front.

It was hard not to imagine, with our having learned that caregivers seemed to divide their time among several agencies, that our rejection of the nurse who wasn't reliable about showing up (Aaron) and the nurse who issued edicts to be followed "or else" (Gretel) had left the folks at Redux with a dilemma. Fortunately, we had a midafternoon appointment with Carlos and his team, whom we could rely on every day except Sunday, but that didn't feel sustainable for the long term.

For this visit, we asked for additional adhesive, since Ben had me up from 3:00 to 4:00 a.m. replacing Monday's special sacral bandage when it became dislodged during a middle-of-the-night bathroom adventure. So Dani and I tried a different technique for situating it so it might be more secure. Not that Ben could tell, but she and I also invested a lot of energy trying to convince each other that progress was being made and that the bedsore was getting smaller.

"It is, don't you think?" She held the measuring tape; I snapped a photo. We looked at several days' worth of images and told each other, "It has to be."

We had yet to hear anything more from the Department of Children and Families. With no idea what legal engagements might be in our future, our only choice was to do our best to get Ben into shape for hip surgery.

And yet I was extremely tired, and Ben's patience was extremely short and his list of demands extremely long. I was deeply disappointed in myself at how frustrated and angry I was over my inability to just "suck it up."

People talk of the need to preserve the dignity of and respect for those requiring care, but I was beginning to obsess over the need to preserve the dignity of and respect for those *giving* care. I was grateful at the core of my being to have Ben home, but he'd begun to channel a self-centered, grumpy, demanding narcissist whose utterances had been stripped of common civility.

"Turn that off."

"Turn that on."

"Grab that. Quickly!"

"Bring those here."

"Take a message"—after I'd raced up the stairs to hand the phone to him because the caller required Ben's direct and immediate input.

When I could find the time, I channeled my frustrations into my journal.

Meanwhile, as Ben's cognitive function came back online, he turned much of his attention to the lakes in the neighboring park and Daniel, the rising college sophomore majoring in marine biology who, during a summer internship, had taken up residence nearby to help care for the lakes' fragile ecosystem. If Ben wanted a change of subject, he'd focus on renting out the cabin up North or preparing his mother's tax returns.

I didn't appear to be on his list except as an extension of his arms and legs, there to serve 24-7 as his chauffeur, secretary, housekeeper, personal servant, dresser, butt wiper, pill dispenser, laundress, and errand girl.

And even as it seemed possible that the Department of Children and Families had shifted the focus of its investigation from me to the home health-care agency (which hadn't been in touch, so that had to be what was going on, right?), the sting and paranoia remained. Was someone watching me? Judging me? Reporting me? Who? And when, for crying out loud, had I become such a fragile, vulnerable, sheltered wimp?

I knew there wasn't supposed to be any compensation for being here and taking care of Ben. He was home with a new heart, and we were safe in a beautiful spot with full cupboards and comfortable quarters and relatively healthy bank accounts, even as it felt like the world was falling apart, what with the pandemic and escalating political battles and the senseless killings that had inspired the ongoing Black Lives Matter protests. I had friends who'd lost their mates and would have given anything for the opportunity—the gift; no, the miracle—I had been given.

And yet my journal had become a litany of unending complaints. What the *hell* was my problem? Seriously—who did I think I was?

I needed to find both my big-girl panties and my bootstraps.

There were so many things I'd rather have been noting in my journal. How enjoyable menu planning and cooking were now that Ben was back to a low-salt versus no-salt diet. How the moisturizing regime Carlos had recommended for Ben's legs and feet (with me seated on the floor in front of him, slathering handfuls of Aquaphor or CeraVe on his parchmentlike calves and ankles) reminded him of the poolside "treatments" he and his sister, at ages three and four, used to give their grandfather when he'd let them smear him with suntan lotion decades ago back in New Jersey. The cornucopia of notes, cards, articles, and emails that continued to arrive from all over. How blessed we continued to be to have so many people keeping him and us in their prayers.

Wednesday. Another early-morning round-trip to the clinic, this time to see the nephrologist. And then a call from Synchronized Basics: Redux would be in touch today. I'd believe it when it happened.

But then at 3:00 p.m., I took a call from Anita. "I'm a registered nurse. I'll be by this evening to assess Ben's case on behalf of Redux." She kept her word, arriving at 7:45 p.m., just in time to be sure Ben went to bed with fresh bandages.

I knew I should be grateful and relieved, but damn. We were only two weeks into his being home, and I was spent. When would I be able to trust that we could win this war?

With the start of business on Thursday, Sasha's supervisor from the Department of Children and Families called to talk with Ben and ask how he was faring, but she couldn't provide any update. And the lawyer called too. He suspected that we'd never know the origin or the final results of the department's investigation. If we found we needed him, he'd be just a phone call away, but he didn't think we would.

Finally, shortly after lunch, the newly assigned Redux nurse, Connie, arrived.

When she departed forty-five minutes later, Ben had fresh bandages for the second day in a row, and he didn't have to leave the house. This was a first, thanks to the home health-care assistance we had foolishly assumed would be a daily occurrence more than two weeks earlier, when he'd been "discharged to home."

That same afternoon we had another FaceTime session with Dr. Giraldo, the pain management specialist. He was pleased to hear that Ben was managing with only one oxycodone pill every twenty-four hours and renewed the prescription to get Ben through the coming month. Noting that the oxys each contain 325 milligrams of acetaminophen, he counseled us to be hyperaware of Ben's Tylenol intake and not to exceed two thousand milligrams of acetaminophen in twenty-four hours, because that might trigger other issues.

When Nurse Connie arrived on Friday afternoon, she let me know she wouldn't be coming over the weekend, but before my heart hit the ground, she continued, "So let me show you how this is done so you can do it tomorrow and Sunday," and as she addressed each of Ben's wounds, she gave me a tutorial and encouragement.

It was Father's Day weekend, which meant several Zoom calls with friends and family. Ben logged on at his computer, while a floor away I logged on at mine, the better for each of us to hear and participate. I ping-ponged between staring at Ben's image, marveling at his being here, taking an active part in the conversations, and being miserably distracted and distressed by how wiped out I appeared. And he spent hours on the phone with each of our boys, listening and laughing and loving every minute of it. As spent as I was, I managed to take joy from that.

The weekend also brought the opportunity to practice what Nurse Connie had taught me, and so long as the bandages were going to be replaced anyway, it was time to brave getting Ben in and out of the shower. He'd been getting stronger every day; we could do this.

I laid out towels, clean pajamas, a laundry basket, a trash can, and a tray holding disposable gloves, saline solution, gauze, the prescribed ointments, fresh dressings, scissors, and tape. Then I set a tub of Aquaphor, more gloves, some paper towels, and a pillow on the floor, where after the shower and the application of bandages I could sit cross-legged and massage Ben's lower legs. After that, I situated the shower chair and set a bar of soap, shampoo, a washcloth, and a back scrubber within reach. Finally, I turned the faucet on to get the water to a good temperature, then I turned it off again.

"Everything's ready when you are. Are you feeling strong enough for this?"

"Yes—it's gonna feel great."

Ben steeled himself, and we worked together to recall the tips Victor had given us ten days previously, maneuvering him over the threshold and settling him onto the chair. He reached forward with the back scrubber, turned on the tap, and relaxed.

From start to finish, it took nearly an hour, and there were some bits to be tweaked before the next effort, but we'd done it—success!

"That was exhausting, but thank you. It's wonderful to be clean. I think I'll take a nap now."

"Are you okay with my going for a walk?" Time spent wandering along the edge of the water and under the palm trees would help ground me and clear my head as to where things stood.

"Yes, go for a walk—I know you want to. I've got my phone; you've got yours. Go. And when you get back and I wake up from my nap, maybe we can go look at that bed."

A couple of days earlier, as he was glancing through our local weekly paper, he'd torn out a classified ad for an adjustable king-size bed free for the taking. It was the last thing needing to be cleared out of a house that had just been sold. It seemed that although Ben was being a champ about not overdoing the oxycodone, he wasn't sleeping as well as he should.

I was skeptical that such a visit would work, but the home was wheelchair-friendly, and the moment Ben saw the bed, he knew he had to have it. With a simple handheld controller, he'd be able to elevate his feet, sit up, or do both—plus every variation in between. In addition, the bed railing we already had was adjustable enough to remain functional. A couple of phone calls later, arrangements had been made to have it delivered to "his" bedroom on Tuesday.

Now he was on a roll.

"And if I had a remote-controlled recliner in my office, I could nap right there without having to go down the hall."

Another phone call, another delivery scheduled. When I mentioned the recliner to a friend, she suggested that perhaps a nursing pillow would be useful as well, as support for a mealtime tray.

As for the existing king-size bed, which was really a pair of twins placed side by side, the furniture delivery team helped me dismantle everything and stack all the pieces (box springs, mattresses, and frames) in one tall, teetering pile on top of a bed in the next room. With the state of Florida setting national COVID infection records, it wasn't like we'd be hosting overnight guests anytime soon.

In the meantime, Nurse Connie had shown up on Monday and Tuesday as promised and had even given us her schedule for the rest of the week and the week that followed, which would lead into Independence Day. I took to working side by side with her during each visit, learning a little more every time. The instructions she'd provided to get us through Father's Day weekend had been a gift; the reliable scheduling moving forward, a godsend.

CHAPTER 15

Adjusting to Our Foxhole

June 23, 2020—July 15, 2020

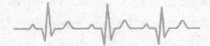

That first shower had been a confidence builder, and Nurse Connie's reliability provided tremendous peace of mind. We'd worked the Aquaphor treatments into the daily schedule and finally were managing successfully to get Ben into and out of the shower every other day. Three of Ben's five wounds were healed and no longer required attention, and the tracheostomy would join them soon.

However, while Ben had hoped that the new bed and recliner would magically rectify all his sleep issues, that was not proving to be the case. And, as many professionals had warned us, the bedsore remained a significant challenge.

Yet over the course of the three weeks he'd been home, a lot had been accomplished. Routines, from meds and daily meals to visits with doctors near and far, had been laid out, and some had even been perfected. I hoped we had finally settled into a good pace for this marathon, even if we had no idea how far we'd come or how many more miles remained.

I revisited the daily schedule I'd drawn up shortly after Ben had been admitted to the ICU at the end of March, hoping to rework it to help us best negotiate being restricted to Florida for the summer—not just by Ben's recovery but also by ongoing COVID issues. Despite the state's declaration that it was open for business, its COVID case numbers continued to balloon. We had no choice but to plan on sheltering in place for at least the next four months.

Given that reality, I then made a list of priorities, with item number 1 being weight—the challenge of putting some *on* Ben while getting and keeping it *off* me. He had gained, maybe, three pounds since returning home, even though he was eating three full calorie-dense meals a day plus desserts and a couple of protein shakes as snacks. But the transplant team assured me that as his medications list and dosages evolved through the coming months, adding pounds would become easier.

I, on the other hand, had been modeling weight-gaining behavior and was up ten pounds, which prompted me to face the question, Who do I want to be when (if) the world settles into a new normal? An important part of the answer was: not someone carrying around these extra pounds. They were bad for my back and uncomfortable in the heat, plus they made it harder to get around and not as much fun to get dressed in the morning. So. That.

Item number 2 was getting organized—including everything from our desks and our closets to the kitchen cupboards. Our home had to suit the way we wanted and needed to live; it could no longer be the patchwork it was because that way had been easiest when we moved in and my back wasn't cooperating.

Item number 3: acknowledging all the emails of support from these past two and a half months, which were still continuing to fill our inboxes daily.

Number 4: staying on top of our finances. I'd mastered a lot of "Russian grammar." It would be a shame to lose ground.

But also, we needed to have more fun than just what playing backgammon and gin rummy offered. Maybe getting out on the water was what we needed. Or learning French (for real—not Russian). Perhaps taking up a needlepoint project would be good for me too.

What was on Ben's list?

Getting a new hip as soon as possible, because with that in place, he'd be able to undergo physical therapy. And with physical therapy, he'd be able to get strong enough to climb into a deer stand. And if he were strong enough to climb into a deer stand, he'd be able to convince all the doctors that letting us head to Pennsylvania for the month of October would not be unreasonable. We could see his mother, our children and grandchildren, and harvest some venison for the freezer too.

Ben grew both more anxious and more hopeful the closer we got to the last Friday in June and his scheduled telehealth appointment with Dr. Manrique. Surely we'd be able to set a date for surgery: when the fracture had been discovered in April, the timeline mentioned for repairing it had been "three weeks after 'discharge to home.'"

In preparation for the session, the doctor's nurse, Jenny, and I went over all Ben's medications and his vitals, then she had me text up-to-date photos of the bedsore for the doctor's reference.

"Oh, and by the way, Mrs. Cart, the doctor is working from home this week."

As the appointment began, Dr. Manrique asked Ben a lot of questions about how much his hip hurt and whether the pain-management guidelines were proving effective and helpful.

"Are you getting enough sleep?"

"I'm working on it. We got an automated bed so I can elevate my legs and sit up more easily or shift around in the night without Sarah's having to come upstairs to help. And a recliner so I can nap here in my office. But it's tough, and it feels like it's getting tougher."

"Well, there's good progress being made on that sacral wound, but it's still not far enough along to schedule a full hip replacement because of the infection risk that comes with the metal prosthesis. You do have some options you can consider, however. The procedure we've discussed before would be a stopgap pain-relieving measure—the one where I would remove the ball of your hip but not insert the prosthesis until a later date when it's safer to do so. By 'safer,' I mean when there's no more bedsore and less COVID in the hospitals. Ultimately, you'd end up with a markedly shorter left leg, and in the meantime, you'd have to get around exclusively in a wheelchair. You wouldn't be able to stand or use a walker for even the minimal amount of time you're doing those things now. Or we could up your daily oxycodone intake, but that will make the withdrawal much more challenging when the time comes."

"No—I don't want to have to go through more withdrawal than I'm already in for."

"Okay. Understood. I know you were really hoping that we'd get you on the schedule for the full replacement, but even if you said yes to the stopgap option today, I'm so sorry to have to tell you that you'd have to wait at least another week. As Jenny mentioned, I'm working from home this week."

There was a pause. He looked like he might cry, then he said, "The fact is, I'm quarantining; I've got COVID."

"Oh, no!" Ben and I were both stunned and concerned. "How are you feeling?"

"Tired. A bad cough. Achy. But getting better."

"And your wife?"

"She's avoiding me and staying healthy so far."

"That's a relief, but oh, we're sorry you're going through this." We struggled to hide our disappointment.

"Me too, especially since it delays things for you, but let's plan on meeting in my office when you come up for your next biopsy. It looks from your chart like that'll be two weeks from yesterday. And in the meantime, I can see you're scheduled to come to the clinic for a COVID test three days before your next biopsy. I'm going to have Jenny make an appointment for you to see Dr. Mascaro. He's an infectious disease and wound specialist and should be able to help move that bedsore along.

And don't be alarmed when you pull up your chart online or see the insurance notes—the wound specialists work out of the plastic surgery department."

He paused, teary-eyed. "Ben, I know you're disappointed and discouraged. I know both of you are. I'm sorry. We'll get that hip fixed, I promise."

With that, all three of us were crying, dispirited by the bedsore, COVID, and the feeling of helplessness.

Over the weekend I began a new three-week meditation series focused on "welcoming change with joy and acceptance." The accompanying commentary emphasized the need to focus on small victories every day and enjoy every change.

My takeaways: Exercise greater awareness of my choices about sleeping, eating, moving, and handling stress. Shift from allowing fear to serve as the primary incentive for change and instead move toward visions of a better life and lifestyle. Be receptive; accept the present moment; allow room for inner peace, a quiet mind, and . . . bliss.

It wasn't as easy as it sounded, and after a weekend of hardly doing anything in the wake of Dr. Manrique's news about having to delay the hip surgery, Ben spent most of Monday in bed in a sad, sulky funk. His pain would not abate, and thus his sleep patterns were reverting to those of six months earlier.

"There's no reason to bother to try to get to my desk. And it's too hot to go outside. Besides, if I don't move too much, it doesn't hurt as much. Maybe if I'm not sitting, the butt sore will get better circulation. I'm just gonna try napping."

Midday Monday, a call came from Redux. Because of insurance issues, Nurse Connie wasn't going to be able to treat Ben again until "the doctors issue new orders, and even if that got sorted out today, she can't visit until at least a week from tomorrow because of the upcoming Fourth of July weekend."

We'd stalled out, and the national news of record-breaking COVID numbers not only in Florida but also throughout the country wasn't helping. Nearly all the political pundits and medical experts were in agreement that it was only going to get worse.

We hobbled forward, one hour, meal, shower, bandage, nap, dose of pills at a time, anchored by appointments scheduled with Carlos and his nurses for Tuesday and Thursday to help with general morale and the bedsore dressings. But at the Thursday appointment, Carlos looked at the wound, raised his eyebrow, and frowned at a new snotty-green discharge.

"I don't like the looks of that." He took a culture and put Ben on antibiotics.

With the holiday weekend looming, Ben's hip had become so painful that too frequently both of us were weepy over our inability to relieve it. He wasn't sleeping well, and the only place he could bear to be was bed. I felt like we were falling down a rabbit hole or caught in a catch-22 spiral.

And then it was Monday again. Time for another trip to the clinic for a regularly scheduled COVID test in anticipation of another Thursday biopsy—Ben's seventh post-transplant. Thanks to Dr. Manrique and Jenny, however, this trip included "an appointment with plastics" to discuss the bedsore. We got on the road midmorning Monday hoping for some definitive direction, advice, and action but not counting on any of the above.

When we got to the plastics appointment, I learned that watching what Dr. Mascaro termed "a full debridement procedure" is, for me, best handled with smelling salts in hand. Ben was a champ and never complained as, with gauze and saline, the doctor aggressively rubbed the ugliest parts of the bedsore raw, then applied silver nitrate and packed some bandages in place.

He also provided me with instructions for replacing the bandages with ointment and fresh dressings as soon as we got home. I asked about the green stuff that Carlos had cultured, but the doctor wasn't too worried; the antibiotics would knock that back.

As I fulfilled my assignment a few hours later, even my untrained eye could see that the bedsore, while not smaller, looked, somehow, better, which felt like a step forward.

Only to be followed over the next two days by several (what I hoped were small) steps back.

First, somehow Ben pulled a muscle in his upper chest, likely as he used the bedrail to maneuver himself into the least uncomfortable position for his hip, and as a result, he was now in excruciating pain any time he coughed or sneezed. Second, the results of last week's culture came back: pseudomonas, the same infection that had resulted in his being put on IV antibiotics in early March, a few weeks before he ended up in the hospital. And third, for the first time in months, he suffered a couple of bouts of heartburn over the course of forty-eight hours—attributable, I hoped, to the antibiotics.

When Ben had pseudomonas the first time, the infection didn't clear up until he was in the hospital and the transplant team agitated to have it addressed aggressively. So at this point, it was hard to trust that a few pills a day taken at home would do the job, but doubt wasn't going to help, either.

At least none of these issues delayed Thursday's scheduled cardiac biopsy—which Ben aced—and another virtual visit with Dr. Manrique. While we were on location at the hospital with Jenny, the doctor was still home, awaiting clearance to return to work. The conversation started with a review of the options: continuing with pain management only or removing the ball joint completely.

But then the doctor presented a new possibility: implanting a temporary prosthesis made of antibiotic-imbued cement. The cement version would not be as large or secure as a permanent metal replacement, but it would last between twelve months and five years—or longer, depending on Ben's body's response. It would require consensus approval from the cardiology, plastics, and infectious disease departments, but it could be scheduled before the end of the month and would require three nights in the hospital, maybe. But then Ben could go straight home without having to stay in a rehab facility.

The surgery would be similar to a full-on hip replacement, for which Dr. Manrique outlined the steps once again: they'd administer a spinal anesthetic if that was okay with the cardiology department's anesthesiologist. There would be an anterior approach. An hour in the OR. Application of the dressing. In recovery until cleared by anesthesiology. Then back to the hospital room and walking that same day.

This time, however, Dr. Manrique followed up with the risks, of which there was a 10 percent chance Ben would experience at least one.

- Adverse reaction to the antibiotic-imbued cement.
- Infection, in which case the doctor would need to either (1) open up and wash everything, then put it all back; (2) replace the cement piece; or possibly (3) remove everything and be done for the time being, leaving Ben in a wheelchair until a metal prosthesis could be installed at a later date.
- Fracturing of the pelvis or leg.
- The hip popping out postsurgery.
- Nerve or blood-vessel injury resulting in numbness at the back of the thigh, which, 98 percent of the time, resolves itself in around three months.

A lot to think about, and pretty sobering, but most immediately, our job was to get the pseudomonas under control ("Jenny, see if you can get them in for another visit with Dr. Mascaro before they head home today") and pray that Florida's COVID situation, which was continuing to deteriorate in record-breaking ways, wouldn't nix the possibilities. Plus continue to work on good nutrition, made more challenging by that morning's blood-work revelation of elevated potassium levels, which changed some medications and meant pulling bananas and ice cream off the menu until further notice.

Jenny worked her magic, and within an hour, Dr. Mascaro was debriding Ben again, and knowing that this was what was delaying Ben's hip surgery, he offered to do the same for us every Monday for a few weeks.

While driving home from the clinic, I reflected on a bizarre sensation I'd experienced that morning as we arrived. Everyone was well masked because of the pandemic, but as I pushed Ben's wheelchair into the elevator, a few staff members looked *so* familiar. My initial thought had been, *Well, we've been coming to the cath lab for over a year*, but then while pacing the hallway an hour later as Ben was undergoing the procedure, I glanced at the signage and realized what should have been obvious: the cath lab was adjacent to the SICU, where Ben had lived for so long.

The familiar faces were the nurses who'd enabled our FaceTime sessions when he was too out of it to do it on his own. I was incredibly grateful to each one of them, especially because they kept showing up even as Florida's virus situation continued to skyrocket out of control.

Having hauled the wheelchair in and out of the car for Thursday's adventure, I woke up Friday with a fragile back and remembered the advice physical therapist Christine gave me mid-March: "Hurt does not mean harm; it means time to rest."

I flipped back through the pages of my journal and came across an entry from early February: "Whenever I can make the time, now and moving forward, I must do whatever I can to nurture the strongest version of me, physically and mentally . . . *focus* and *execute* . . . Need to emphasize *joy* and *gratitude*, *grit* and *grace*, rather than fear, lost time, or loss."

With the tantalizing suggestion of surgery before the end of the month, the biggest challenge of caregiving for Ben had become standing by, powerless to alleviate his hip pain, and being the bad cop who, when he was finally in a relatively pain-free position and getting some desperately needed rest, had to wake him up for time-sensitive meds. The worst was administering the magnesium pills, which were hard to swallow and would start disintegrating the instant they touched his tongue, coating it and making him want to cough or gag. If he were lying down, he wouldn't want to sit up because doing so was too painful, so he would make me put the two pills in his mouth and pour water in after. He'd struggle to swallow because he wasn't upright, and the water either trickled down his chest or choked him as I accidentally filled his mouth with too much. I despised having to do that because he would swear and cough, and water would splatter all over his shirt and the bedding. It sucked.

At least when I had to play bad cop and put him through the ordeal of a shower and rebandaging, his mood would improve with the post-shower calf and foot massage I gave him.

Dr. Mascaro was supportive and encouraging when we returned for the next appointment.

Good progress was being made: the one huge wound had broken up into two smaller ones.

Interestingly, he didn't believe the sores themselves were infected—they just needed to be aggressively cleaned, to the point of rawness, daily.

"You're the one who put this bandage on yesterday, correct?"

"Yes."

"Then you can do this. Just wash your hands, put on some gloves, and do what you've watched me do here. When you finish up, make sure the bandage keeps the two wounds separated. It'll take time before these heal completely, but they'll be far enough along to avoid delaying any surgery beyond the timetable Dr. Manrique has laid out. Keep up the good work, and we'll see you next week."

That was all well and good for a Monday, but come Tuesday, Nurse Connie, whose orders had been renewed immediately after the July Fourth weekend, was quite distraught. She didn't want to hear about any plastic surgeon's suggestion to "clean more aggressively" because "that's not in the orders." We didn't have anything in writing from Dr.

Mascaro, and her job was dependent upon her following a doctor's written prescription to the letter. She would rather quit than get fired.

I tried explaining that we hadn't been making as much progress as we should with the methods employed so far—and then crossed my fingers and hoped that when the dressing came off on Wednesday, she'd see that we were on the right track.

The bedsore did look better on Wednesday, but ugh and dammit—for weeks, Ben had not taken the lead on his meds. So when I was on a late-morning walk to the market to grab a few items, he texted me to say he was going to take his antibiotic. "Okay?"

Immediately I texted back: *"No!"*

Response?

"Oh. Well. Already did."

I'd given the antibiotic to him less than an hour earlier; he'd been all caught up. And now he'd doubled the dose. *Crap. Crap. Crap. Crap. Crap.* Because more diarrhea and losing additional weight was such a great way to build up his strength for a hip replacement.

As for me: I needed to double my dose of joy, gratitude, grit, and grace, STAT.

CHAPTER 16

Enduring Together

July 15, 2020—August 8, 2020

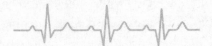

O ur days had grown busy, busy, busy. I'd prepare a breakfast tray (juice, coffee, hot cereal, and applesauce, or French toast and sliced mango, or pancakes and a peach, or scrambled eggs and toast, or a bagel and cream cheese—and, almost always, a banana milkshake, except when we'd been cautioned not to overdo his potassium) and give Ben his morning meds.

An hour later, his antibiotic.

An hour after that, a shower (on the days when he could muster the energy) and a dressing change.

Late morning, more meds.

A lunch tray: soup and a sandwich; or reheated leftovers (he's never been a big fan of those); or, on the days when the pain was up and he was a bit down, a plain old peanut butter and jelly sandwich made with unsalted peanut butter. Plus a protein shake and/or a refreshing, cold glass of a fizzy vitamin C dietary supplement. Then, for dessert, pudding, Fig Newtons, or applesauce with vanilla wafers or graham crackers.

Midafternoon: more meds and a "treatment"—massaging ointment into his calves, ankles, and the tops and bottoms of his feet to keep the skin moist and intact.

Dinnertime: a full-on well-rounded meal, with maybe an ice cream sandwich, carrot cake, or banana bread for dessert. And more meds.

Bedtime: an antibiotic and more meds.

But the progress was slow, and always in the back of my mind, I would hear the drumbeat of "hurricane season preparedness." We'd never stayed straight through the summer and fall before, partly because rainy season in the Keys begins in May and ends in October and because hurricane season technically begins on June 1 and runs through Thanksgiving, with its height being in August and September. As summer progresses, whole weeks can be consumed with watching a system develop phase by phase as it decides what track to follow while residents determine whether they have everything needed to shelter in place. That means stocking an emergency supply (three days' worth) of food, water, and medicine plus flashlights, extra batteries, nonperishables, important documents, personal identification, and, if applicable, pet food and fuel for a generator. While I already had all that covered, true preparedness also means having an exit plan ready in case the authorities declare a mandatory evacuation.

To that end, the moment Ben arrived home in June, we had sprung for a one-year membership in a small private aviation club. If we were told to leave, "all" we had to do was get to one of the several small airports in the Keys or on the mainland just west of Miami. The representative who'd sold us the membership promised that, although we'd likely be sharing the flight with others, they could get us out of south Florida to someplace safe with just a few days' notice. And at least Savvy could be with us in the passenger compartment and wouldn't need to be crated. But I'd wake up in the middle of the night fixated on how I'd manage to get her and Ben, her bed and food, and all his medical equipment to the designated airfield. Then I'd obsess over how they would get Ben aboard without causing him excruciating pain. I didn't want to borrow trouble, but we had to be prepared.

Then, just when we least expected it, on a seemingly random Thursday, Dr. Manrique called on the landline. Ben took it in his office while I listened on the extension in the kitchen.

"Change of plans: What's on your calendar for July 31? Wanna get a hip replacement? I've talked this through with several of my colleagues. If you're up for it, the risks are not high enough to warrant implanting a temporary rather than a primary prosthesis. I'll work my end, getting all the doctors on board, if you'll work yours—calling those doctors and persuading them to agitate on your behalf for insurance approval." We were also to continue with the daily ministrations and prayers to move the bedsore along.

Ben refused to count on it, and COVID could still derail the whole plan, but it gave us something to focus on. I allowed myself the luxury of imagining what a wonderful thing it would be for Ben to have no more pain in his hip and to finally be able to cherish the gift of his new heart. Then I concentrated on fostering gratitude and hope, even knowing that we needed to play all this close to our vests. Should the plan fall apart, it would be easier to handle the disappointment, bitter as it would be, by ourselves, without having to soothe other people.

For the next fifteen days, we would take things sixty minutes at a time—and we knew many of those minutes would be long, because at this point, Ben's pain was driving almost everything, including his diminishing appetite. At the rate he was going, he'd weigh around 140 pounds on his way into the OR. He took to napping a lot; I hoped that would change when his hip finally was repaired.

After a month and a day, the home health-care situation was starting to fall apart in slow motion. Nurse Connie arrived one afternoon reporting that the contract needed to be renewed again. To that end Ben immediately sent an updated photo of the bedsore to Redux. Within an hour, the insurance company called to report that Redux was shorthanded.

"Nurse Connie is no longer available," I was told, which was odd, because she'd said, "See you tomorrow" on her way out the door.

"Would you like us to pursue finding a new agency?"

With a slew of upcoming appointments at the clinic and the requirement that for the five days leading up to surgery Ben take daily showers with a specially prescribed soap—which meant I'd likely be the only one on hand to apply new dressings—we said, "Not now. We'll probably have new orders after the surgery anyway. Let's wait."

But the next morning, Ben received a text from Nurse Connie: "Hi, Ben. On my way. See you in half an hour."

Problem was, twenty minutes earlier, I'd taken another call from the insurance company, which was wanting to verify our decision to hold off on any additional care for now, since it had reconfirmed with the Redux folks that they remained shorthanded. "The nurse is on vacation," the representative told me. Wires had crossed somewhere, and we were about to get Ben into the shower.

Eager to follow the doctor's orders with that medicated soap, Ben opted to press on rather than text back just then. But as it happened, Nurse Connie never showed up. Maybe she'd decided after all that she was entitled to take that vacation the insurance company claimed she was on.

At least, thanks to Dr. Mascaro's silver nitrate ministrations and tutorials on debriding, great progress had been made on the bedsore.

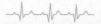

As the days went by, Ben's growing nervousness about going back to the hospital came to permeate every interaction. He obsessed about the pain in store for him, how hard it was to get any sleep in the hospital, the impossibility of getting any privacy in the bathroom, and the specter of ICU delirium. Such obsessing was uncharacteristic for him and unlike anything he'd ever shared with me before. Either the worrying was new or his ability to hide it was gone.

One night I lay awake imagining how the various dynamics would shift once Ben was on the proper side of this broken-hip issue. At the point when we found ourselves in some post-COVID world, one in which we'd be allowed to travel and get back north, our friends and family would have already established new ways of getting along without us.

And closer to home, once Ben was able to enjoy being on the road to recovery for *real*, what would *that* look like? How would *our* dynamic evolve? He'd been really sick for a very long time. How would he trust that he was healthy again? How would *I* trust that? How healthy would he be? Could we posit faith that the systemic sclerosis would take a major pause?

And having had to lead for so long, while admittedly having relaxed pretty quickly and completely when it came to letting Ben take over again at his desk and all that meant for managing our household finances, at what point would I step back into simply being Ginger Rogers? That is, following Fred Astaire's lead but doing it backward and in heels, as they say?

With one week to go until the operation, we had Ben's pre-op consult with Carlos. One box checked. Each of us was thinking a lot about how everything would play out. Ideally, in seven days Ben would be home, recovering from surgery, and on his way to much less pain and much more control of whatever pain remained.

We counted the hours—they moved slowly, and we did too. Although the days were warm and humid, in many ways the heat was easier to bear in the Keys than it was up North. Here the temperature remains steady and stays in a narrow window—in the eighties all day and all night—while Miami and Fort Lauderdale are both much hotter, a combination of all that concrete and being farther from the water. We reminded ourselves that we were in the northern Caribbean (perhaps not technically, but we might as well be) and took what small comfort we could from embracing the lifestyle and mindframe of the tropics, wearing lightweight clothes and not hurrying to get anywhere.

Lying awake that night, reminding myself to breathe, I imagined I was on vacation up North now, a guest in Jillian and Pete's home, on the edge of beautiful Sebago Lake, with loons calling in the distance and Ben sleeping soundly and comfortably in the other bed. Who knew if or when we'd ever get to do that again? "May it be soon. May everyone be safe. May the next 168 hours be full of victories, success, joy, and gratitude."

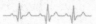

Monday morning brought lots of red tape and numerous phone calls. There was the social worker setting up post-op physical therapy. (Based on our experience back in June, I could only marvel at her optimism.) There was the surgery coordinator, who said we still needed the nod from cardiology, and the transplant coordinator, who was still waiting for insurance approval. There was the pharmacist, to remind us to pick up refills the next day when we came for Ben's pre-op COVID test. Then the transplant coordinator again, regarding scheduling next month's refills. Then once more, the surgery coordinator, who scheduled a cardiology visit during the next day's visit to the clinic. Finally, there was the transplant coordinator yet again, rescheduling that cardiology visit as telehealth, since an in-person visit would have taken place after the COVID test, and once Ben had been swabbed, he was to stay home until being admitted on Thursday.

In the meantime, there was breakfast to be prepared, pills to be administered, and a shower to be taken, complete with a pre-op cleanser, a dressing change, and leg "treatments."

On Thursday morning, the surgery coordinator called: insurance said no to Ben's spending the night before surgery in the hospital, so surgery would be at 2:00 p.m. Friday instead of first thing that morning. Also, Ben was to remember to bring his walker. Meanwhile, I tried not to obsess over the news that Tropical Storm Isaias was predicted to travel through Florida "sometime" Saturday, and no one could say how long after surgery Ben would have to stay in the hospital.

My journal entries for the day of the surgery and the eight days following tell the story.

July 31, 2020

Sitting in the CCF cafeteria. Surgical coordinator called late yesterday afternoon: Could we be at the clinic by 8:30 a.m.? Uh, yes. Although it meant I had to drive the two-lane road out of the Keys against rush-hour traffic at dawn, it also meant that Ben could still benefit from some residual late night pain relief. He was to have nothing after midnight—he'd been dreading that insurance would say no to an overnight stay, and thus he'd have to endure the trip with no medication, so early surgery is a bonus. Hopefully it also means that the end of the day falls into place a little more easily. Friday evening traffic to the Keys is usually wretched, but with Isaias promising a windy, rainy weekend, at least most of the people on the road will be residents.

Whether our car will be holding one resident or two remains to be seen.

Check-in was at the same desk as biopsies and cath lab, so all feels reassuringly familiar.

Only glitch is that, because they are "expecting lots of patients this morning," all caregivers have been asked to find other places in the hospital to wait, at least until midday. So I am here, having turned in my coupon for a complimentary cup of coffee, noshing on some expensive cookies, mask-free. But the mask will go back on shortly, and then I will pace the halls waiting for my cell phone to ring with the news that he's out of surgery.

Let's go, Ben—please find your way back to me again.

August 1, 2020

Ben's HOME!

I have to keep pinching myself, and I have a stupid shit-eating grin that won't go away. There's plenty left to pay attention to: his temperature, blood pressure, bedsore, medication schedule, etc., etc., but did I say? He's HOME!!!

Exhausted, but HOME.

Bless Dr. Manrique and all the CCF folks who took care of him yesterday, and Dr. Manrique again for calling late last night to be sure we'd made it home safely despite the weather.

Ben's HOME! Thanks be to God.

August 4, 2020

Isaias passed southern Florida observing social distancing guidelines, thankfully, and is now raining its way from the Carolinas through Pennsylvania, heading into New Jersey, New York, and New England this afternoon.

Ben's recovery is more painful and slower than he had hoped, which has had him down for the past couple days, but he did start physical therapy at the medical center yesterday.

Hopefully his spirits will pick up as he starts to move a bit more.

Sadly, one casualty of Isaias was the small bonnethead shark who had been residing in the reflecting pool in the park—too much wind sent the brackish water over the banks, too much rain meant too much fresh water, and the change in salinity meant there was too little live bait left for him to eat. Ben has taken the loss hard.

August 5, 2020

Yesterday Ben went off on a solo exploration via golf cart, having strapped his walker to the side, for the first time in over 130 days, which he found both exhilarating and exhausting. I wish he were as enthusiastic about eating and gaining weight, although I know that will come.

His second PT session was today, and the therapist pushed him twice as hard as she did on Monday, so he's napping with an ice pack now. He's still waiting for his guts to kick into gear reliably, but that's not likely to balance out until he's off the painkillers. In the meantime, in addition to the postsurgical pain, there is some postsurgical swelling, but oddly, as I see it, the swelling just makes him look a little healthier—we need to accept progress however it presents itself. He still weighs barely more than 150.

August 7, 2020

Waiting on two telehealth appointments in a row—much more convenient than driving all the way to the clinic, but the timing is always risky, since they get to you when they get to you.

Hopefully, the two different departments won't get to Ben at the same time.

Took an excursion to the optician's yesterday so Ben could get an eye exam and a new glasses prescription, which he's needed since the end of last year. Funny how it kept falling to the bottom of the list. I'm sure vision issues added to his dementia and compromised capabilities in the SICU both before and after the transplant.

Time passes so strangely. Ben's hip surgery, a week ago, feels like it was just the day before yesterday, maybe because he's only now getting around as well as he and we had hoped he'd be doing 48 hours post-op. Three PT sessions under his belt. He reports these four weeks (three remaining) will be focused on learning to walk and balance properly again. He is taking the pain meds more often and more regularly, thanks to Dr. Manrique's explaining (he's been wonderful with follow-up phone calls) that now is the reason Ben was moderating his dosages through June and July—so that the meds would still be effective when he really needed them.

But the other side of that coin is that he's sleeping a lot (because of meds and PT) and not always thinking as clearly as he had been. Kinda like he's drunk, but without slurring his speech, and since he's not yet fully capable of walking, he doesn't give away the status of his capabilities by weaving or losing his balance. So. Need to be aware and wary of his judgments. Not really an example, but he did not appear for breakfast as we had agreed he would only 20 minutes earlier. When I went to check on him, turns out he was having a gut-clearing episode in the bathroom.

"Are you okay?"

"Oh, yes. My stomach doesn't hurt as much anymore."

"How long has it been hurting?"

"All day yesterday. All night too."

"Were you going to mention it?"

"Didn't I?"

"Nope."

August 8, 2020

He's doing better every day, although the going is s-l-o-w.

Stuck in a weird time-space loop these days: COVID/ transplant/summering down South rather than up North. Startled to get emails re: planning for Labor Day even as it still feels like April/May. Ben lost many weeks while he was in the hospital, and apparently, I lost them too.

We've got everything we need for a fresh start (heart, hip, house)—except energy and momentum and real time-space awareness.

And yet there have been experiences removed from time, like enjoying the fruits from our garden even though we didn't invest in their beginnings—mangoes, limes, star fruit, figs, Surinam cherries—and doing hurricane prep, realizing, even if this isn't the year for it, that we can and should flow back and forth more easily between North and South throughout the summer and fall.

More immediately, over these past many months I've focused a lot on gratitude because that was what sustained me, but right now I'm feeling the weight of the ongoing burden of responsibility. He's *so* close to being back, but he's not completely there yet—the marathon's still on, and it's exhausting, getting him to appointments, administering meds, layering on the calories, managing the calendars . . . and there's grieving to be done and indulged in (briefly) regarding all that COVID has robbed us of: time, humanity, people's lives and livelihoods, progress. The soul-crushing politics.

I have no illusions: we have been incredibly, miraculously blessed, but I miss our kids and our grands and our friends up North and the ones from down here who managed to get away for the summer. I miss hugs and handshakes and seeing people's smiles and laughter and tears mask-free.

I need to get back to head-clearing swims in the mornings and walks later in the day as soon as Ben is well enough. And while I may have to produce numerous calorie-ingesting opportunities each day, the task has been made easier because I've been able to split and freeze many of our meals, and Sarina and others have been fabulously generous, dropping by delicious dishes at least once a week. Plus, while Ben still has to be careful about salt, those restrictions have eased up considerably since he got his new heart, so the options have broadened.

CHAPTER 17

Stutter Step

August 8, 2020—September 7, 2020

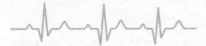

All was well and good until our community medical center's doctor on call reached out midafternoon on Saturday. When I answered, I had déjà vu: this was too close to the conversation I'd had with Carlos on March 27: "Sarah, I'm looking at Ben's newly arrived results from blood drawn on Thursday. His hematocrit is dangerously low. Whom are you supposed to call at the clinic when he has a medical crisis?"

I had no idea, since this was our first over-the-weekend who's-on-call crisis since Ben's return home, more than two months earlier. She wanted a name and phone number and fax number so she could forward the results and have someone on his team take responsibility, because "this isn't good and can't wait. People have strokes or heart attacks with this issue."

She had my attention. "Let me try the phone numbers I have, and I'll get back to you as soon as I have some answers."

I put in a call to the transplant coordinators' line, since they were the ones always calling with test results. After a long time on hold, the answering service passed along a message: "You need to talk with his cardiology team."

So I tried a different number and was put on hold for another long time before being disconnected.

Finally, I took the whole issue to Ben, who'd been napping most of the day. Was that because he'd been exhausted by the previous day's physical therapy? Or was it the meds? Or . . . was it the dangerously low hematocrit?

He used his phone to try getting through another way and succeeded in reaching cardiology's answering service; he put them on speakerphone.

"Oh, you need to talk with the transplant folks"—at which point I took over.

"No! We tried that already, and they told us we had to talk with you. Please! The local doctor on call has made this sound like a life-threatening emergency. Who's on call there? Who can help? Whose phone number can we give to this doctor down here in the Keys before she goes off call for the night?"

"And you are?"

"This is Ben's wife, Sarah. He can't hear you well enough because he's having issues with his hearing aids."

"How about I track down the cardiac nurse for you? Someone will call you back."

While we waited for that callback, I passed along a fax number and the list of clinic cardiologists' names to the local doctor.

Fortunately, the cardiac nurse did call. It was Sophia, who had called me on Easter to let me know that Ben was back on "the list." To extricate us from the middle of the communications about this current crisis, I asked if she would please call the local doctor directly, pointing out that the medical center is not an urgent-care or emergency facility, so its Saturday hours would be drawing to a close in around thirty minutes.

Then: radio silence.

Nothing from CCF. Nothing from the medical center. A less than relaxing evening.

At eight thirty Sunday morning, Sophia called back to ask how Ben was doing ("I think he's okay") and report that she'd spoken with the front desk at the medical center twice late yesterday afternoon, but the doctor hadn't been available and didn't call her back.

In the meantime, however, she'd been able to access the test results, which she agreed were screwy. She advised we get them run again in case they were in error.

"Just go to your nearest ER."

"But our medical center doesn't have Sunday hours. The closest ER is forty minutes from here, and in light of COVID I'd rather drive all the way to the clinic so he's being looked after, with all his medical records right there."

"I understand. Since he seems to be doing all right, if you want, you can wait until first thing tomorrow," but as stressed as I was, eighteen hours into this fright, I really did not want to wait and then subject myself to the drive against early-morning rush-hour traffic.

"How about you think about it and talk it over with Ben? I'll give you a call in half an hour."

When she rang back, I told her that Ben and I agreed that a Sunday drive, with light traffic on a beautiful day, made more sense to us than waiting another twenty hours. It had already been seventy-two hours since the blood draw, and if the hematocrit was getting worse, waiting wasn't going to help.

We packed up his phone and his meds for the day, plus his walker (no wheelchair!), and arrived at the clinic's ER at 11:00 a.m. But the masked security team stopped me. Now that Ben was able to enter using a walker rather than a wheelchair, I wasn't going to be allowed to enter the building with him. Together, Ben and I explained that he wasn't going to be able to hear well enough to check himself in: they obviously had reservations, but they kindly made an exception.

Once check-in was complete, we settled in to wait, but when an aide came to take him back to an exam room twenty minutes later, the security guards stepped up and told me I had to leave the building.

So I walked. And walked. And walked. In the shade to the north of the hospital.

Meanwhile, Ben texted me several times as they worked him up for COVID, gave him an EKG, took X-rays, and did all new blood work. The hematocrit results were going to take a while, however, because that sample needed to go through a centrifuge.

At one thirty, when Ben asked for his lunch meds and pointed out that he was going to need magnesium at three o'clock, the nurse told him that although the test results were not yet visible in his chart, she could see doctors' orders that he was to be admitted. They'd prescribed a blood transfusion, and they still wanted to determine whether perhaps there was some internal bleeding. I was furious with myself: each of the dozens of times I had taken him to the clinic in the two months since he'd come home in early June, I always had his go bag with me: phone charger, iPad and charger, extension cord, nail clippers, a change of clothes—but not today.

Having only the phone with which to say good-bye, I left him with 70 percent battery power and his optimism that a nurse would let him borrow a charger. Then I drove home. As much as I despised the predawn drive against the weekday commute on our two-lane road into the Keys, it was nothing compared to 3:00 p.m. on a summer Sunday. The last twenty miles were terrifying: people passing across the double yellow line. Everybody speeding. Hard-to-see bikers scooting in and out. Trucks blocking visibility, hot rods, crazies, horns. But I made it to home sweet home and found the house eerily quiet. Savvy tucked her tail to her belly and refused to leave my side.

I hoped this would just be a quick overnight. Not an impossible thought, right? Even the hip surgery had ended up being an outpatient procedure—proof that hope didn't have to be in vain.

I reread the last few entries in my journal and realized that, on some level, I should have expected this. Ben had not been himself. I should have said something during the week, before everything slowed down for the weekend. I should have made some calls, trusted my gut instincts, and recognized those instincts for the advanced warning system they are. I needed to learn to *speak up sooner*.

I began Monday with an early-morning swim to clear my head, then took a long time running errands (groceries, post office, banking) before heading back to the hospital. Perhaps these were unnecessary delays, but each was a task that needed to be accomplished, which might mean that I (and, I hoped, Ben) would return to a more organized home front at the end of the day.

As a result, much to Ben's frustration, I didn't arrive at the hospital until noon, but then felt so blessed to be permitted to go to his room. He'd been experiencing bad PTSD, what with the sights and sounds, bright lights and beeping monitors, and the comings and goings of techs, nurses, doctors, custodians, and other phenomena reminiscent of March, April, and May. When I finally walked in, however, he took comfort in being allowed a visitor and having access to the chargers for his phone and hearing aids, plus his razor.

The hematocrit was better, and the doctors hadn't found any signs of internal bleeding. In fact, they'd been hoping to discharge him, but there was a glitch: they needed a stool sample.

They'd timed their request badly, registering it ten minutes after he'd emerged from the bathroom, so he was working on that, while I worried that poor Savvy was probably at the opposite end of the spectrum at home, desperately needing to go out and trembling as thunderstorms approached from the west. And even once they got the sample, we were still going to have to wait for a doctor to issue the discharge orders.

Yet the delay was providential, because a wound nurse came in to check the bandage on what remained of Ben's bedsores. She talked with me about all the various ointments and asked what we'd been using most recently.

"Oh, at this point, you need to stop using that prescription. It helps generate new growth, which is why these ridges are starting to develop. For now, you should just use the MediHoney. You'll be done with these soon, and congratulations to you on that. I first started working on this in May, back when there was just one huge butterfly, before he got discharged to rehab. That bedsore was one for the record books."

Her hands-on instruction for wound care might have been worth the price of this hospital admission.

Ben got to eat dinner on hospital time (4:30 p.m.), then finally they let us leave. He slept for the long drive home as daylight faded, and after a joyous reunion with Savvy, went straight to bed. His conversion to the hospital's schedule continued the next morning, so I gave him an early breakfast, and he followed with a post-breakfast nap, during which he and I agreed I could get in a swim.

The hematocrit episode left us with a new wound care routine and a new nutritional goal: iron-rich foods as well as renewed attention to eating proper meals on a regular schedule.

But the regular-schedule part demanded teamwork, and on Tuesday, I completely lost my temper. Having prepped and delivered his lunch tray and after-lunch meds to his office at twelve thirty as he worked at his desk, I returned at three with his magnesiums, which were not to be taken in conjunction with anything else.

His lunch—and meds—sat on the tray untouched. "Aw, c'mon, Ben! Are you kidding me?"

"Okay, okay! Calm down. I'll handle this. I'll finish lunch and those pills now and take the others in an hour."

When I returned at five to spirit away the meal tray, he was surrounded by paperwork and focused on his computer, barely having touched his lunch. All the pills remained where I had put them.

"Why the hell do I bother?!?"

"Wha—" He jumped, not having heard me come in.

"Dammit, but you make me mad! Why do I keep taking the trouble to sort pills, make meals, change bandages, renew prescriptions, schedule appointments, drive and drive and drive and drive, and so much more, if you're not going to do your part? Which in this case was pretty damn simple! How *dare* you!"

Ninety minutes later, I was silent as I served him his dinner on the porch. "I'm sorry. I just got lost in projects at my desk."

His words hung between us as neither of us ate.

Finally, I sighed, "It's not fair, Ben. Yes, this is all about you, and right now it has to be. I get that; I'm living that every day. And I'm amazed and grateful that you found your way back to me. But the reality is, you still have a long way to go until you're well enough and strong enough to do the things you say you want to do. You obsess about getting back to Pennsylvania for a visit this fall and being reunited with all the friends and family we've been missing for so long. Those are things I want to do too. Desperately.

"In order to do that, however, you need to focus on making a full recovery, and you need to be safe, which means you need to eat right, sleep right, and take your meds. You've come such a long way, but you're nowhere near recovered yet. You're still toe-touch weight-bearing— you're not even walking yet. And even without the world's COVID craziness, the clinic's transplant protocol means you can't travel until mid-October at the earliest. According to Jon, in Hartford, it's one year of 'stay-close follow-up' appointments—and that's *before* recovery from your hip replacement gets factored in. *You* have to do your part."

I stood up and cleared the table, leaving Ben sitting quietly and somewhat abashed, staring at the park's palms, poincianas, and tamarinds silhouetted against the evening sky as he considered all that had been said.

Still, despite the hospital stay, Ben *was* making tremendous progress in physical therapy, even as he needed to learn to walk again—plus stand up, sit down, and navigate the stairs. And, thanks to this same hospital stay, daily progress on the healing bedsore was clearly visible to the naked eye.

In addition, because of the hospital stay, over the course of the following week he had another follow-up appointment with Carlos as well as a previously scheduled follow-up with Dr. Manrique and a telehealth session with the nephrologist. Between all those meetings and his newfound independence, his renewed obsession with the neighborhood park and its lakes, and his determination to do whatever it might take to get north in late October, day-to-day life was getting notably busier and notably more exhausting.

We were living the miracle but doing so required constant discipline and single-mindedness and attention to detail. Which is why the start of the in-person checkup with Dr. Manrique stunned both of us.

"You were admitted to the hospital on Sunday and didn't call me?!" He was bereft. "I could have helped! From here on, keep me in the loop. Please!"

The truth was that we, Ben's doctors, and the whole cardiology team had been so focused on Ben's being a heart transplant recipient that his having just had hip surgery hadn't occurred to us as being in any way related. Yes, the hip surgery was all over his chart for everyone to see, but in neglecting to reach out to Dr. Manrique and his partners, we'd missed the fact that it's not unusual for hip-replacement patients to experience low hematocrit levels postoperatively; the orthopedics folks could have helped shed light on the situation.

Phooey.

The conversation turned to the primary purpose of the visit: how Ben was doing with the new hip. Dr. Manrique was glad to hear that Ben had finally understood and come around to increasing his use of the opioids to better manage the pain sustained in the wake of several grueling hours in the OR.

"It's time now, however, to start weaning yourself off them and using acetaminophen instead. I will not be giving you a new prescription. And you will not be getting any more from any other doctor."

Ben's eyes opened wide as he absorbed what that meant.

From there, Dr. Manrique instructed Ben to continue to use the walker and refrain from putting his full weight on the left leg for another month. He explained that this was to keep the implant in place. Otherwise, the additional pressure would make Ben's left leg much shorter than his right.

It felt like Dr. Manrique was holding something back. Finally, and most heartwarming for us, he shared his elation at how well Ben was doing two weeks along. "You're my first post–heart transplant guy!"

As he escorted us from the exam room, he proudly called his colleagues into the hallway to watch Ben "walk" out. "Doesn't he look great? I am so proud of you, Ben. And you too, Sarah. You're doing an awesome job."

From that appointment I drove Ben into downtown Key Largo to get fitted for his new glasses, which were to be delivered in a week or two, and then home for another meeting about the lakes, this one with a horticulturalist whose expertise was Keys flora and whose knowledge of Keys fauna was not far behind. Ben was making huge strides and getting back into his element. A full, busy, and productive day.

At bedtime that night, I found Ben sitting on the edge of his fancy bed, with its comfort-providing remote, counting his pain pills.

"If I were to keep taking them at the rate I'm taking them now, I have enough to get through mid-September. Let's see if I can get off of them before Labor Day."

"We've got a good supply of Tylenol on hand; just let me know what you need."

The following day included another lakes confab, a meeting at the park manager's office, and a physical therapy appointment, all of which Ben went to by himself, taking along a packed lunch and his meds. He also got the first of two pneumonia vaccine shots, administered by Carlos's team as directed by CCF.

For my part, I welcomed this dawning of a transition. I facilitated the smoke and mirrors necessary for all those meetings to go as smoothly as possible, but too, I'd managed to get to the pool five days in a row. Progress on many levels, for both of us.

Way to go, team!

And as proof that Ben was receptive to new tricks, when I delivered his lunch on a tray to his office on Saturday, he dropped everything to eat it in a timely fashion.

It was almost as if he'd seen my crib notes anticipating his "I want to rent an RV and go to Pennsylvania" sales pitch, expected any moment. Weeks earlier I had nipped such a conversation in the bud, saying he was in *no* shape for us to discuss such an undertaking because he wasn't even walking yet, and I would have to do all the heavy lifting plus 99 percent of the driving.

I'd ended with, "Let's not talk about it until at least the Glorious Twelfth," a reference to the annual August 12 opening of grouse season in Scotland, long ago added to the family lexicon because it was also his sister's birthday. But since the Glorious Twelfth happened to follow immediately after that fateful day when he'd so thoroughly pissed me off by neglecting to eat his lunch and take his pills on time, he hadn't dared raise the subject of traveling anywhere.

Still, I knew it remained front of mind for him when one of the doctors ratted him out during the course of a busy week: "Say, I hear you're wondering if and when we'll let you travel. My nurse mentioned you're hoping to rent an RV to go north in October." Oh, how I wanted to avoid arguing with him about this.

As Ben's next cardiac biopsy approached, we were blessed with one significant change: up to this point, every biopsy required that a COVID test be performed at the clinic seventy-two hours beforehand. That procedure had been modified, however, and the clinic would now accept a COVID test from our local medical center.

Despite that improvement, being able to address Ben's medical needs from home had its frustrations. Since the transplant, four months previously, my cell phone number had been the one provided to every one of Ben's doctors. The thinking behind this was obvious at first, and as the weeks passed, it continued to make sense for several reasons. I was the one managing the calendar and therefore scheduling appointments, so it was logical for the various doctors' offices to call my number to confirm them. I was the one who could hear a phone ring. And when it came to telehealth, Ben wanted me to be part of the conversation, taking notes and repeating things for him that he couldn't hear.

One Monday morning in mid-August, he was scheduled for a 9:00 a.m. telehealth follow-up with the nephrologist who had overseen getting those stubborn kidneys back online in May.

Typically, someone from the doctor's office would call first, and we would review Ben's medications list. Then a short time later, the doctor would call. But this time, there were issues getting a good connection. First, I answered two calls to find no one there. Ten minutes later, I missed a third, because when I needed a bathroom break, I'd left the phone with Ben, and even though the ringer was set at its loudest, he didn't hear it when it rang.

Because Ben was the one the doctor would need to talk with, and I didn't want to risk answering the call elsewhere in the house only to lose it while running up the stairs, I was stuck waiting in Ben's office.

An hour went by. Then another thirty minutes.

Attempting to placate me, Ben observed, "Well, at least we didn't have to drive all that way!" (Note that he hadn't driven anywhere all year.)

I knew he was right and things were going miraculously well, but my fuse was short. I couldn't get a walk in or go for a swim. Couldn't run errands. And, apparently, I couldn't leave Ben unattended trusting he would answer my phone if it rang. So I had to sit in his office and wait. At least I could read on my Kindle while doing so. We did manage, finally, to have that appointment, and we were relieved when it didn't reveal any major issues. Afterward, I took my self-pitying sulk to the pool for a mile's worth of laps.

Then, just as we were getting relaxed about being able to handle medical tasks close to home, Ben took the golf cart out for an evening fishing adventure—just a man, his walker, a fishing rod, and a couple of lures to throw from the breakwater. But upon his return, unbeknownst to me, he neglected to plug in the golf cart's electric charger. So the next day, when the time came to go to the medical center for some blood work and a COVID test—foolish me—I thought I'd drop him off and run a few quick errands in the neighborhood.

No such luck. The golf cart barely got us to the lab; I wasn't sure it would even be able to get up the slight grade at the entrance. And I *really* didn't want to roll backward into the street. In the end, we made it, and on time, but I drove straight to the nearest electrical outlet, at the back of the building, and made Ben hoof it, walker and all, around to the front. Once the vehicle was plugged in, I stayed in the parking lot to pace off my extreme frustration—under the trees, in what little shade was available.

Splat.

Water? A fair amount of it, despite a cloudless sky. Strange . . . and a couple of tablespoons of it had landed on my head. Ah, phooey! I stepped aside to look up into the branches, wondering what kind of bird could produce so much pee.

Splat! This time the liquid landed on the pavement, which was fortunate, because it was a large, poopy green mess. Then *splat* again, right next to the second one.

Finally I spied the culprit, but I couldn't imagine why it took me so long. Mr. Iguana, well over two feet long, was gawking down at me through the leaves, giving me the one-eye, and if his posture was any indication, he was quite pleased with himself.

Seeing him reminded me that the previous afternoon I'd caught sight of a beige house gecko running across the rug in our bedroom. I wondered where it had ended up and wished that Ben would move back into our room. Surely a joint gecko catch-and-release adventure would ensue—I with a glass and a piece of cardboard to slip underneath while Ben opened doors so our house guest could be freed outside. It would be a reversal of our usual roles, but it would also be a spirit-lifting and welcome echo of past shared escapades.

The iguana was a wake-up call: I may have been going a little stir-crazy as Ben pushed the limits on his returning sense of independence, but considering all the twists, turns, and battles of this journey, I couldn't imagine a better outcome.

We were so lucky, yet we were also getting cranky. It was rainy season, which means many days are all about waiting for the thunder and lightning and moisture to move through. Unlike the usual pattern up North, however, the typical sequence of events in southern Florida is that once the storms pass, the air often becomes an even warmer and heavier wet blanket than it was before. At such times, I was finding getting out to walk or swim for any distance an impossibility. And as thrilled as I was to have Ben making great strides, there were moments when he'd annoy me so much that I just wanted to bop him on the nose. Meanwhile, he was taking to throwing mini tantrums when I delivered his lunch: "Fine. I need to drop everything and eat this *right* now, or it won't get done."

Plus, the mail wasn't always as reliable as I wanted it to be, which meant that critical and expected, but late, package deliveries (of Ben's prescriptions, for example) would frequently have me on edge.

It seemed while Ben would stress whenever he was at his desk, I was stressing over every other detail in our world, from the little stuff at home, the tropical weather, and the threat of COVID to the issues across the country and around the globe: unemployment, racial unrest, climate, and politics.

It was 2020; I was not alone. *We* were not alone. And "we" were "we"—what more could I ask for? What more could we possibly want out of life?

Arriving just before 7:00 a.m. on Thursday, August 20, for biopsy number 8, we came through the hospital entrance at the same moment as Dr. Manrique, who was beaming at having just watched us maneuver our way across the parking lot. Yes, we'd come from one of the handicap spaces, but we still had to walk a good distance. We'd become such regulars that the familiar faces, from the guards at the door and the clerks at admitting to the cath desk receptionist and the nurse who took Ben back to the lab, commented one after another on how wonderful and amazing it was to see him enter *on foot*. He was using a walker, but he was moving under his own power and with strength and energy. Bless them all.

Once the procedure was underway, I solved the ever-changing mystery of where the seating for the cafeteria had migrated to as a result of the hospital's ongoing construction projects. This time, as I settled into a far corner with my laptop and calendar, I found myself marveling at "how we spent our summer vacation."

There had been dozens of doctor appointments, reminiscent of the chaos at the start of the year, but they were tapering off, and while the earlier ones had been crisis-based, these were wellness-focused. Except to maneuver into his bathroom, Ben had spent all of June and July in his wheelchair, but after his hip replacement, although he was still toe-touch weight-bearing on his walker, he was getting around on his own. He was also making mischief. Damn golf cart battery! Damn inconvenient mealtimes! Damn rumors about his scheme to travel in October!

I sent up a prayer to all those spirits I'd implored to stand by his head, his heart, and his hip when he was deep in his darkest hours upstairs in this building. I knew they remained right there with us, just as they had been months earlier. And I knew they were amused that he was up to a little trouble again and, on occasion, annoying me.

And it was wonderful.

I headed back to the cath-lab waiting room at the appointed hour, and soon Ben ambled in with his walker.

"Hey there, Mama Cart! You wanna take me home?" Yes. Yes, I did.

This was a seismic shift from the times when the nurses would send me off to bring the car to the hospital entrance, then wait for them to wheel him out. The moment they appeared, I would jump out of the driver's seat and work quickly with them and the security guards to transfer him and load up his wheelchair and various go bags, rushing to get out of the way of whoever needed to do the same next.

We walked back to the car, together, and headed home.

Daily attention still needed to be paid to the wound at his tailbone. He had miles to go before he'd be able to put weight on his leg, and he was having a few GI issues, likely attributable to withdrawal from the pain pills, but there was a palpable sense that we were finally approaching the mopping-up stage of our battle plan.

Again, way to go, us.

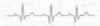

In the wider world, Tropical Storm Laura was lashing the southern coast of Puerto Rico and heading our way. We could only pray that she, like her cousin Isaias, would practice social distancing as she cut through the Lower Keys en route to the Gulf of Mexico, where she was likely to do some sort of interesting tango with Hurricane Marco (the weather folks were all excited by this unprecedented dual storm development). And a new tropical depression was forming off the western coast of Africa.

We'd need to stay mindful, but I finally felt confident that if we were told to evacuate, getting Ben and Savvy onto a plane would be manageable. It might be unpleasant, but we'd get it done if we had to.

As we kept an eye on the weather over the second-to-last weekend of August, Ben complained that he was having trouble getting to sleep at night. I reminded him of his pre-Christmas appointment with Carlos during which they had discussed Ben's sleeping habits.

Carlos's "prescription" then had been sensible and sound advice: "You'll be better able to function during the day if you get a good night's sleep. Go to bed at eleven. If you aren't asleep by eleven thirty, get up and read until you're sleepy. On the first morning, get up at four thirty. On the second morning, get up at five; on the third morning, get up at five thirty."

And there were rules. "*No* television, computer, phone, or iPad after 9:00 p.m., and *no* naps during the day."

Ben was frustrated by my reminder. But then on Monday, at physical therapy, his therapist advised him, "Stop taking naps at all hours during the day!"

A thirty-to sixty-minute afternoon nap still made sense—he was weaning himself off a powerfully addictive medication, after all—but going back to bed immediately after breakfast felt extremely counterproductive. So on Tuesday morning we played cards—he beat me soundly, even though he could barely stay awake; harrumph. And for the rest of the week, he took over the dining-room table to work on a jigsaw puzzle whenever he was tempted to sneak off and lie down.

Putting away some laundry for him on Thursday, I realized he'd hidden away the rest of his oxycodone. Out of sight, out of mind . . . progress.

Way to go, Ben.

As for me, I'd been working obsessively on a Christmas needlepoint project, hoping to pull off a miracle and finish it in time for the needlepoint shop to do its part to complete it—cleaning it, blocking it, and turning it into a velvet-backed stocking for our oldest daughter-in-law. If only I could master walking while stitching. But at least while I was stitching, I couldn't be eating!

Jigsaws? Needlepoint? We were living a life of leisure . . . miraculous.

Then, at bedtime the Saturday night of Labor Day weekend, before getting on the elevator to go up to "his" room, Ben noticed a strip of light under the door leading from the house to the garage.

"I wonder what that's about. Oh—*oops!* I'll bet the bougainvillea hedge blowing in the wind is tripping the motion detector out there. Klutzy me—I left the garage door open. That's not great for the air conditioner."

Having listened to Ben's thought process, I watched as he maneuvered himself into the garage and hit the button to close the door before returning to board the elevator. We said good night, and I listened to the elevator creak upward as tears welled in my eyes.

For the first time in well over a year, it felt as if there were another responsible adult living under our roof.

Yes, he'd been wonderful about taking back the reins on all kinds of office and paperwork projects, touching base with bankers and insurance companies and utility providers, and he'd been hard at work coordinating the marine biology intern and the horticulturist and various projects to improve the health of the lakes in our community, but on the home front—getting to and from appointments, running errands, preparing and cleaning up after meals, coordinating with contractors, locking up at night, and all the other stuff that makes a household run—I felt as if it had been all me for months on end. Not a lot of teamwork.

Until the garage door needed to be closed so the air conditioner could do its job.

All I could do was say, "Thanks be to God and the universe" for having sustained me and us through some unbelievably long, terrifyingly dark days.

Monday, September 7
Labor Day Ben report

Hi, all—

It's been a long time since you've heard from us, but take that as proof of the adage No news is good news.

Ben's new hip has made a world of difference in smoothing the road to recovery, even though that road is still long. It is a tremendous relief to have the excruciating pain from his July 31 hip-replacement surgery behind him—different but much more manageable than the pain from the broken hip itself. With good guidance from the pain-management team, Ben was motivated to detox as quickly as possible after his three months of dependence on painkillers. Thus we are happy to have June, July, and August in the rearview mirror and grateful that storms Isaias, Laura, and Marco all practiced proper social distancing on their way by the Keys. We're hoping that any cousins that may be spawned over the next couple months prove similarly polite.

Everything to do with Ben's new heart continues to meet everyone's highest expectations.

With the hip surgery, he graduated from wheelchair to walker, and PT at our local medical center, five minutes away, has been miraculous as he learns to walk again. Two weeks ago, he found a way to strap his walker to the golf cart so he can get himself there and back on his own, fabulous for restoring his sense of independence and mine. After his appointment with the hip surgeon tomorrow, he hopes to be allowed to put his full weight on the leg (although "full weight" is a very gener-ous term—he's barely 150 pounds sopping wet) and maybe even swim. It's been a couple years since he's been in a pool.

In the meantime, a friend shared a Clint Eastwood quote the other day. The iconic movie star was asked how he continued to make movies at his advanced age. Apparently, he said gruffly, "I don't let the old man in." A plan we are adopting immediately, even though we seem to have lost almost all track of time. If you woke either of us in the middle of the night and asked, "What month is it?" we would both probably tell you that it's still April.

During this strange-for-us summer in the Keys, we have been fascinated to learn what blooms when, whose mango trees produce fruit
the longest, and where the Key limes are. We're also eager to discover
whether that bunch of bananas just around the corner is ever going
to ripen and thrilled to taste the Surinam cherries, Key limes, and figs
from our own yard, while all around the neighborhood, we find lots and
lots of avocados.

After a long spring and summer focused entirely on Ben's health, just
in the past couple weeks he and I have begun to realize it might be safe
finally to envision a time "beyond." We're even discussing a road trip
north for a few weeks in October if the doctors give their blessing.

xoxoxo SAC

CHAPTER 18

Balancing Act

September 8, 2020—October 16, 2020

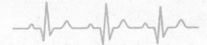

The day after Labor Day, we made the trip to the clinic, and I stepped up to sign Ben in at the orthopedics desk while he took a seat in the waiting room. When I turned around, I realized he'd settled into the lowest couch in the room.

"Are you serious? What were you thinking? They've got all these automatic recliners that will stand you right up when the time comes—and you opt for a couch?"

"I wanted to have room for you to sit beside me." Making mischief. How annoying. And adorable. Sigh.

A few minutes later, Dr. Manrique came to get us. When does that happen? It's usually—no, always—a nurse.

"Ben! Sarah! Let's head back to the exam room."

I stood up and looked back at Ben, frustrated for myself and embarrassed for him that he was going to have to struggle to get himself out of a jam, but he simply grabbed hold of his walker and rocked forward, trying to move his center of gravity. Then he rocked a second time, and finally, on the third go, he got enough forward momentum to stand up. Dr. Manrique gave him a huge smile.

And then took the walker away from him. "How about you lead the way?"

Ben headed through the door and down the hallway, while the doctor and I fell in behind. As we followed, Dr. Manrique leaned toward me and said softly, "Watching him fight to stand up like that just now told me everything I need to know about how well he's recovered from the surgery," and then as we passed a nurse's desk, he reached out and grabbed a box of tissues. Not until he offered them to me did I realize I was crying. I had not seen Ben walk unassisted for more than five months. It was a beautiful sight.

And although he used his walker to get back to our car, once we arrived home, he officially transitioned to a cane—the one he'd bought back in March, when his hip first hurt.

The day after that, we were scheduled for a phone meeting with a Social Security representative because Ben had realized over the summer that he could file a disability claim. Shortly after I arrived in his office with my laptop, calendars, and all the spiral notebooks in which I had logged the questions and answers from every doctor's appointment and every phone conversation since November of 2016, the representative called.

The plan was for the conversation to take one hour; instead, it went on for nearly two and a half, during which we provided the names of and contact information for every doctor, the date of every diagnosis, the dates of Ben's first and most recent appointments, and much more. Ben said he'd learned the week before that his Cleveland Clinic Florida "abstract" was more than eight thousand pages. The representative was stunned at the volume of information and said she'd submit his application for review soon; a decision would be forthcoming in a few weeks.

But while so much had been going right recently, we had one more battle to wage, this one between us. As mid-September approached, there was no way to avoid Ben's intense desire to get to Pennsylvania ASAP and stay for as long as possible. In our attempts to avoid all-out war, negotiations were tense, partly because I couldn't imagine that what terrified me about being in the Poconos—COVID, distant medical care, box-store grocery shopping, short dark days, and *no* possibility of social interaction—wasn't blatantly obvious to Ben. He was hyperfocused on his wishes and wants, yet as miraculously well as he was doing, he was nowhere near fully independent yet.

Making the situation even more challenging was the reemergence of Ben's lifelong ability to put a positive spin on *anything*, including the cautionary email Sophia Wilson, in her capacity as the head transplant nurse, sent to the whole team when she heard the rumors of the Poconos plans: "While Ben is doing as well as we could hope, with his autoimmune issues, he was not a typical transplant patient, and his has not been a typical recovery . . . delayed hip surgery . . . hematocrit episode. A complicated case."

"Did you see Sophia's email? She didn't say we couldn't go!" Awkward.

I was on edge, knowing this was not going to go away until we had it out. As we sat down to dinner one evening, he set his cane on top of the table, with its rubber-tipped end right by my place setting.

"No! You *cannot* do that." In a snit, I picked the cane up and moved it so it was leaning against a chair at the far side of the table. "I do not want the end of your cane, with whatever it may have picked up from wherever you may have been—your office, the yard, your bathroom—anywhere near my meal. Thank you."

Although he led with "I'm sorry," there was tangible pushback. "The cane is new to me. I'm still learning where I can put it, because it doesn't stand up well when I lean it. I need to figure out how to manage it."

"Perhaps my point would be clearer if I were to remove my shoe and place it next to your place setting. In fact the issue is not what you do with your cane but rather your awareness—or lack thereof—of how your actions affect others. You can accuse me of having said this before if you want, but apparently you need to be reminded that this existence we are working through right now is *not* all about *you*."

"So this is about more than the cane."

"Yes, it's about more than the cane. I know you've been counting on a trip north, and that's what's driving your dedication to physical therapy, but I cannot see any way that we can responsibly and safely get to and from Pennsylvania."

We didn't come to terms that night, and not much more was said.

For at least a decade, we have joked that, on occasion, all Ben hears when I speak is the "Mwup mwup" of Charlie Brown's teacher. Indeed—in order for it to register, my message just needed to come from someone else.

When our third son, Ted, called him a night or two later to catch up, Pennsylvania was the only thing on Ben's mind. They talked at great length about what our going there would entail and all the mechanics of such a trip, for us and for others.

Ben explained that he'd be safe. His heart was good; he had his meds; I knew how to feed him; he'd be alone (i.e., not in danger of exposure to COVID) when out exploring in the Jeep or while sitting in any tree stand or ground blind; and we would socially distance from whichever family members could make the trek to come see us.

But Ted got Ben's attention by asking whether he and I could live with any potential consequences. After listing the collection of miracles that comprised our year, as he had done for me months before—my not having to have back surgery, the new wheelchair-accessible house, the heart, the hip, everyone healthy and still employed—he went on, "You'd be pulling all of us out of our COVID-safe bubbles and potentially exposing yourselves to the virus on the road. So you manage to rent an RV: What if you have a breakdown or a medical emergency that demands attention out in the middle of nowhere? Would your making this trip really be 'best practices'? Is making the trip the smartest thing for you to be doing right now?"

Hearing Ben's side of that conversation, I had a eureka moment. For weeks, we had danced around the concept of having a "window of opportunity" to make such a trip, but as I listened to him talk with Ted, I realized that our definitions of that window were a universe apart.

Ben's window included all the time between the cardiac biopsies scheduled for October 1 and November 12, which left October 2 through November 11 for getting to and from Pennsylvania, settling into our cabin, and engaging in every available hunting option from the moment of our arrival until the moment of our departure.

Mine didn't open until October 16, six months to the day post-transplant, and it closed again before November 3, Election Day. Within my time frame, the task was a surgical strike north to see family and maybe some friends, followed by our return to our safe Keys bubble, where all our support systems were in place.

At breakfast the next morning, we touched a bit on all of the above, then retreated to our separate corners.

By evening, he'd emailed me. "Let's think about enjoying the month of October together right here. We have plenty to work on, and to enjoy, as we make our plans and rebuild our lives and our relationship, working our way out on the upside of these amazingly challenging last two years. I love you."

Which was lovely and reassuring, except that within twenty-four hours, he cc'd me on his email acceptance of an October 29 appointment with the Scranton cardiologist. I was confused, and dammit, I was infuriated. I hit Reply to his cc and typed simply "WTF?"

Because we each had several projects demanding attention, by unspoken mutual agreement, the subject of Pennsylvania was shelved.

On Friday, September 18, we headed to the clinic for an appointment with Dr. Elzawawy. What a long three and a half years it had been since that first rheumatology appointment, with its diagnosis of systemic sclerosis—there was a *lot* to catch up on. Because we were running late, I dropped Ben off and went to park the car; I was going to be allowed in, since the COVID restrictions were now based on the state's positivity rates, which were enjoying a brief dip.

As I scurried back across the lot, I took a call from our contact at Social Security: Ben's application for disability had been approved. I knew he'd be pleased to hear that; maybe it would ease the tough conversation we still needed to have about our travel plans.

Our time with Dr. Elzawawy felt like a social visit. Although he'd been the first to prescribe an immunosuppressant, that same drug was now one of Ben's mainstays, as it is for most transplant patients, and the cardiologists would be the ones to dictate Ben's dosages from then on. And while Ben had sustained a lot of damage from systemic sclerosis since the initial diagnosis, except for occasional bouts of Raynaud's, all appeared calm for now. Dr. Elzawawy congratulated us on our endurance through Ben's journey, and we thanked him for all he'd done to ease our way from the earliest months. Moving forward, if and when Ben needed to see a rheumatologist again, it would be as a result of a referral from the cardiology team.

On the way home, I proactively confronted Ben's painful desire to finalize plans to rent an RV and schedule our travels north, starting by pointing out that, just as I was doing right then, I was the one who would be driving. I was always the one driving—except for around three hours sometime back in 2019—and I couldn't imagine being comfortable driving an RV, by the way. Plus, after the year we'd had—the year the country had had—there was no way that being back in that cabin, even though we loved it, was going to be anything but exceedingly different and weird. Not to mention that we'd received a warning from Jon to avoid mold. Ideally, before Ben walked into that space, he said, everything should be deep-cleaned—the bedding, the curtains, the contents of his closet and bureau, all the woodwork. And we were still sleeping in separate bedrooms, for crying out loud—how were we going to room together in an RV?

There wouldn't be some magically exponential strengthening of Ben's legs or energy-boosting cure for his restless sleep or anything remotely normal about road-tripping up the East Coast and back again in the midst of COVID. We needed to wait for vaccines to be approved and administered, still two months distant at best. Finally, I pointed out—besides COVID, the heart transplant, ongoing recovery from hip surgery, and many many many highway hours—there was the attraction of the improving weather in Florida, with temperatures and humidity beginning to fall and birds migrating through. I didn't want to miss October in the Keys.

Saturday morning, I found an email he'd sent me late Friday night: "Agreed for now . . . for a week, if people ask, we will tell them that Pennsylvania is not in the cards this year and we'll see if we still feel that way in a few days. If we don't, then we can change our minds back again."

It was not a definitive step forward, but neither was it a step back.

In the eleven days since Dr. Manrique had allowed Ben to dispense with the walker, he'd made awesome progress relearning how to walk. Soon he'd be going up and down the stairs, and when he'd gained some strength, we would return to Dr. Manrique one more time to have Ben fitted for a lift to compensate for the fact that his left leg was slightly shorter than his right.

As Ben reveled in his freedom, I began to look forward to a shift on the spectrum back to friend and life partner, but I was a little ahead of him. Even as every day he was pushing the edges of his newfound physical independence, he was a bit slow about taking responsibility for the other elements critical to his making a full recovery. If I stepped in to make sure he was getting up in time for his morning meds or taking them at the appropriate times later in the day, he'd take offense. My pushback was to point out that he wasn't the one sorting the pills or taking the calls from the nurses with updated dosages or following through with the adjustments in each day's pillbox.

And I was still feeding him, because left to his own devices, which I'd tried for a lunchtime or two, he wouldn't eat, or he wouldn't eat what he was supposed to. He had no right to be mad at me just because yogurt, which he hates with a passion, was prescribed to counter what-ever the ongoing issue was with his gut.

Slow progress did continue, however. Ben returned from a physical therapy session pleased to show off his ability to go up the stairs one step at a time, leading with his right foot and catching up with his left, and down again, this time leading with his left and catching up with his right ("Up with the good; down with the bad"). A few sessions later, he remastered taking one step right after the other, left, right, left, right.

Deservedly proud, he returned home to declare, "Look at me, taking 'reciprocal steps'!" I had to laugh at his delight.

And yet, as we became more proactive about letting everyone know we were *not* going to be making the trek to Pennsylvania, he started to become more distant. It felt like he was investing more energy building his relationships with the naturalists and the landscapers working on the park and lakes than he was in rebuilding his relationship with me.

Indulging in a bit of self-pity, I told myself it was *not my fault* that COVID (not to mention Ben's health) had imposed severe restrictions and limits on our lives. I so wanted to be appreciated rather than resented, seen rather than invisible, included rather than ignored. Continuing to wallow, I decided the only time he seemed happy to see me was when I could cheerlead his PT accomplishments or provide a signature or a password.

That's how I was feeling as we prepared to settle in for a Sunday evening Zoom call with Pete and Jillian, Dan and Hitomi, and Jon and Carrie. Around twenty minutes before the call, I went into Ben's office to suggest that we call from the same computer, but he explained that he still hadn't figured out how he could wear the headset he needed in order to hear while simultaneously allowing me to hear the regular audio, so I'd have to be on a separate computer. So while the six of them were all together at a rental house on a lake in Massachusetts, having tested themselves and quarantined ahead of time, Ben and I were miles apart.

Swallowing my disappointment, I retreated to my office to click on the Zoom link while Ben wrote a quick response to an email from his mother regarding our travel plans, a "Well, we might not be coming" wishy-washy message on which he cc'd me. Unfortunately, during the lull while I waited to be admitted to the call, I made the mistake of reading that email—so I felt (and looked) gobsmacked when the session went live and throughout the balance of the hour visiting with our friends.

Hadn't we just agreed twenty-four hours earlier that we were going to tell people for the next *week* that Pennsylvania in October wasn't happening?

Which is what I asked him when I stormed into his office thirty seconds after everyone hung up.

As he excused himself to address what we'd euphemistically come to call one of his bathroom emergencies, I pointedly followed up with, "And how would you handle something like that while you're up in a deer stand?"

"Fine. We won't go."

Had I won? It sure didn't feel like it.

A new day dawned. The late September weather was gorgeous, with a light breeze and noticeably lower humidity, but Ben and I were now tiptoeing gingerly around each other.

With the decision not to travel finally made, I worried that he would lose the incentive to do his physical therapy exercises, since he didn't have a deer stand in his immediate future. Late that afternoon, he admitted to being exhausted and having no energy, and I confessed to being emotionally wiped out. Much as I had fought against it, I, too, was deeply disappointed we couldn't make the trek.

Several neighbors had asked us to join them for a socially distanced dinner, outside, that night; all I could hope was that getting out and visiting with people in person would ease the sting for both of us.

It did somewhat, and we were both profoundly grateful for our friends' entertaining conversation and their patience with us, but we were wounded warriors.

As the last weekend of the month approached, I was sorely lacking in motivation to tackle my to-do list, and whatever was wrong with Ben's gut, it wasn't improving. I was jealous of our distant friends and family, who shared stories of their careful and repeated reunions, visiting with one another and their children. I felt left out even as I wondered how in the world we'd ever thought going to the Poconos was going to be a good idea.

And, as if reflecting my mood, Ben's get-up-and-go had gone. Thankfully, he wasn't backtracking, but his progress was just so slow . . .

The way things were going, would we ever be roommates again? We'd each become deeply entrenched in our ways, and it wasn't as if he was remotely interested in anything physical. The therapy exercises wore him out so much that a hug, or even holding hands, felt like too much to ask. I told myself that at least I didn't have to worry that I'd soon be feeling deserted while sitting in our Pennsylvania living room agonizing about him out in a deer stand somewhere while I huddled next to the fireplace—cold comfort.

And yet. After everything we'd been through in the past four years, what a luxury to be able to snip at each other, sulk, and retreat to our separate corners. We had so much for which to be grateful.

A few nights before his scheduled October 1 biopsy, Ben had been up late working on a new jigsaw puzzle. I was startled to roll over and find him standing in our room. By my side of the bed.

"Is everything okay?"

"Yeah. I just thought that after all the nights you've tucked me in over these past four months, I'd return the favor."

He kissed me on the forehead.

"You know, if you moved back in here, you wouldn't have to do the stairs as often."

"That's what I was thinking."

And with that, he was sleeping in the master bedroom again for the first time in nearly a year. Although he needed to get up frequently, he was much less restless, and if we could just figure out how to quiet his GI tract, maybe he'd be able to rest for longer stretches.

Soon, no longer continually attuned to the baby monitor, I was sleeping more soundly and for more hours at a stretch than I had in months.

Thursday morning, October 1, found me doing desk work in the clinic parking lot, since COVID restrictions were back in place and Ben could now walk in under his own power. As a result, he went solo to his "senior osteoporosis" appointment and, we hoped, his inaugural "regularly scheduled" (that is to say, once a year) endomyocardial biopsy. He had a new insurance policy due to begin that day, but it remained to be seen whether, once the business day began, insurance would preapprove the procedure. We'd arrived at 7:00 a.m. for his blood work appointment, after which he got himself to rheumatology to talk about his bone health as I listened in on the phone.

"The concern is why a relatively simple fall at age sixty-one resulted in your breaking your hip. And you say you used to be six feet tall?"

"In thick socks, but yes."

"And you're now 156 pounds—" Yay! Progress!

"—and five foot eight. Some of that is because of the hip, but most of it is because of bone loss, likely a side effect of all your medications. There are things we can do to increase your bone mass. Diet is part of it—you need to get plenty of calcium at every meal—and weight-bearing exercise helps. We'll start with vitamin D and keep monitoring you for now. Then once the cardiac team backs off on some of your other meds, we'll get you started on Prolia injections every six months."

It was a plan; that was good.

And insurance weighed in regarding the biopsy: that was a go, which was also good. I settled into my "mobile office" and made some headway on my desk work until Ben called.

"Hey there—are you offering rides to Key Largo?"

"Why, yes! Yes, I am. How did everything go in there?"

"Great." (Confirmed two days later by the OR result.) "And they gave me a prescription for getting my gut tested, so maybe all that can get resolved."

With our calendar more open (read: "empty") than expected, I began working on long-distance ways to observe Halloween and Thanksgiving and Christmas. Although hopes were high for approval of a COVID vaccine sometime soon, it probably wasn't going to happen in time for holiday travel. There was a slim possibility that Benjamin and Anna, who'd moved to North Carolina six weeks earlier as Anna began graduate school, would come for a socially distanced visit for a day or two at Thanksgiving, but the more we discussed it with them, the more the long drive sounded unwise. So for now the best I could do was plan to send off cards and boxes of cheer across the miles.

Other than that, however, I sorely needed to generate some "Way to go, me!" moments for my mental health. And my joy at the lower humidity a couple of weeks earlier had proved premature. The weather had turned positively soupy again.

A few days later, I ferried Ben back to CCF, this time for a final follow-up on his hip and a newly prescribed annual skin exam, and worked from the back of the station wagon once more as Florida's COVID numbers remained elevated. At least I'd figured out that there was a decent restroom at the gas station just up the road. And he and I both were grateful for CCF's practice of allowing patients who arrive and sign in early to see the doctor relatively quickly, which meant that Ben's second appointment, set for after lunch, was completed by noon. At a minimum, that was limiting the risk of heatstroke for all the caregivers like me who found themselves consigned to the parking lot.

Bonus: the appointments went well, although we were going to have to wait for some lab work. Maybe they'd finally figure out what was causing his abdominal issues.

In the wake of one last hot, rainy weekend, the weather finally broke—a big seasonal change accentuated by visibly shorter days. And midweek, a diagnosis of Ben's GI issues finally arrived: C. diff, which he'd had in the hospital back at the end of April. No wonder Ben was exhausted. The antibiotic had to be specially ordered, which took some time, and insurance wouldn't cover the cost, plus a scary potential side effect (among several) was total hearing loss . . . so we were in for a long ten days of prayers. But we were glad, finally, to have an answer.

After so many crazy months—no, years—it was time to find our balance. COVID treatments and vaccines were almost visible on the horizon, and like the world around us, we were approaching a new normal. But whereas for the world, the new normal felt like a heightened state of stress—upheavals in health care and economics, societal shifts and geopolitical earthquakes—for us, as we continued to shelter in place in our velvet-lined gilded cage, this new normal felt unreal and almost, well, lazy. Yes, Ben had some bone loss and a significant hitch in his step, but he'd been on a hero's journey, and his struggles had given us a fresh perspective. The larder was full, he and I both were finally getting some sleep, and when we were awake, our attitudes were improving.

On October 15, the meteorologist on our local TV station announced that according to her calendar, it was the official end of rainy season, and then she immediately apologized for the fact that the weekend's forecast was for all rain, all the time.

As predicted, it was raining when we woke up on Friday, October 16, but that was of no importance to us. What was important was that it was the six-month anniversary of Ben's transplant.

And he'd found his way back to me.

As the weeks passed, the pelicans returned with the change of the weather—and out-of-state license plates showed up in Florida. The days got shorter, and each night the sun set a little farther south on the western horizon.

The one fig left on the tree in the yard stayed green for ages. When it finally ripened, the birds got it before I could notice. Two of the four banana plants eventually sported a flower and two dozen or so cigarette-size fruits.

The changes prompted me to reflect: Over the course of Ben's illness and recovery, how many times did I cry?

Countless times when meditating, thinking of better moments to come.

The day he went on the list.

The day he was taken off of it.

On Easter, when after the spiritually significant three days, he was placed back on.

The day Benjamin and Anna's wedding invitation arrived, complete with a note indicating that the event had been put on hold because of the pandemic, and then again the day they got married anyway because they'd been looking forward to that date for so long.

When Jessica announced, "There's news. A heart has been allocated."

After hanging up with Dr. Brozzi after he called to say that the transplant operation had been a success.

Numerous times during the week when we couldn't seem to arrange for competent home health care.

The day Dr. Manrique said the infected bedsores meant that Ben was not yet a candidate for surgery and that he himself had been diagnosed with COVID.

Then the day Dr. Manrique told us he was willing to schedule Ben for hip surgery: the light at the end of the tunnel.

The day Dr. Manrique watched and smiled as Ben stood up in the waiting room and walked down the hall without a walker or a cane to the examining room.

And so many, many times when friends and family reached out in ways small and large to help me and us keep it together.

William Reflects

I am so grateful that my parents are both still here as I approach forty. I am very lucky. I also feel like I know them better and love them more than I ever have. I respect them more as individuals and as a couple too. I admire the life they built, and I am grateful for the safe and beautiful childhood they gave me and my brothers. I think I always was, but I can see it more clearly now.

Benjamin Reflects

One of the biggest lessons I learned from the experience of confronting my father's mortality is just how fragile everything and everyone really is. In the same year that I almost lost my father, the whole world ground to a halt. The economy collapsed, and everyone was terrified of getting sick.

The entire experience proved to me that my parents were the people I knew them to be: resilient, caring, and kind. It made me appreciate the fact that they're here for me and always have been whenever I needed them.

As I remembered the tears, I realized how large a role Ben's failing health played in our lives for so long, though we struggled mightily to stare it down, rectify it, deny it.

At the worst, we were so close to it that we couldn't see the magnitude of the situation.

Or is it that we refused to see it? A version of Clint Eastwood's not letting the old man in? Maybe that's resilience.

I love you, Ben. Thank you for finding your way back to me.

Ben Reflects

After having been through this ordeal, I try to do something nice for somebody each day. I was a nice guy before, but I was focused on my business and my children and making sure we had enough money for retirement. Going through something like this health crisis was the first time a force almost wrecked me. So I have a different appreciation for life now.

My medical crisis taught me to not sweat the little stuff. I work very hard on that. Life's too short: I did not come back to life to do things that are not meaningful to me. I also try to do something nice for myself each day. I didn't do that before. Little things—like, I give myself a whole hour and a half to slowly wake up, read the paper, and do whatever I want to do. I try to avoid stress, and I'm much more focused on enjoying my life with Sarah. What can we do now? What time do we have left? Once you get a peek over the transom, you realize that life is not going to go on forever.

Postscript

CAREGIVING

As another spring dawns, Ben's and my calendars look like they've been used for paintball target practice, but thankfully, the commitments are mostly social, with only occasional medical checkups. His miracle is mind-blowing, and his progress continues. He'll be taking immunosuppressants for the rest of his life and is still taking north of 140 pills every seven days, but his energy has returned. He's sleeping less and getting out more. While medical glitches surface occasionally, in the wake of COVID and our past few years, most are minor, and they are fewer and farther between.

Having missed getting to the Poconos in the summer of 2020, we are grateful to have returned to our twice-a-year shifts in latitude. When we hit stress points, we try to slow down, change gears, and give thanks for what sometimes seem to be the simplest things, having learned too well that some challenges go unseen by others. We remind ourselves of those challenges by observing, "Look at you, doing reciprocal steps!" Ben is back to his Tigger-like self, and whenever the opportunity comes up, we dance, mostly a swing-based jitterbug, shamelessly.

Those who watch but don't know us often compliment us on the joy we display; those who've known us for years and know that Ben nearly died watch and rejoice with us.

Years ago, Ben and I adopted an expression we'd heard while fishing for salmon: they strike the fly "just when you least expect it!" That's how the role of patient and caregiver arrived in our lives: just when we least expected it. No partner plans on becoming one or the other until it happens and, inevitably, their shared journey is redefined.

The marriage vows in *The Book of Common Prayer* cycled through my brain like a mantra: "For richer, for poorer, in sickness and in health." As the months passed, those words evolved into deeds, even as I was terrified of losing my best friend, my love, and the shared future we had imagined.

While it was new ground for us, I know people have been dealing with this from generation to generation; it is part of the natural order of things. Nearly every lifelong loving relationship ends with some variation of this theme, and I had notable role models to emulate.

I'd watched from afar as my dad cared for my mom until her death in 1986, after thirty-eight years of marriage. At the time of Ben's transplant, my dad was doing the same for my stepmother, his wife of more than three decades. In 1997, my sister's husband lost his multiyear battle with cancer, leaving her a forty-six-year-old widow with two young children who had health challenges of their own. And not long before Ben's issues grew to include congestive heart failure, my brother was diagnosed with lymphoma and succumbed within less than a year, but with the blessing of his wife and their grown children by his side.

I cannot listen to the song "One Last Time," from the musical *Hamilton*, without tearing up and thinking of the grace and determination my loved ones brought to their fights.

On the most basic level, in 2020, I understood it was Ben's and my turn. Yet being a caregiver, especially during the six months posttransplant, proved the hardest thing I'd ever had to do.

Ben Reflects

I am the first to say that my recovery was harder on Sarah than it was on me. I have a scientific brain. I thought of my physical problems as chemical and plumbing issues. I knew I was with God, that I was right with myself. I didn't have any huge regrets. I was ready to face whatever came, even death.

But what my physical problems were doing to Sarah was very painful. I hope her writing this book is part of her healing and may finally give her closure. Every time an ambulance goes through our neighborhood, Sarah's face reflects the stress of it. In a sense, her recovery has taken much longer than mine. And she can't yet let go of the fact that she was responsible for my every move and that she had to save my life. I realize how fragile her recovery is. In short, what she's been through is so much worse than what I've been through. All I have is a limp, but she has the mental trauma.

No one knows how bad caregiving is until you get stuck with it.

My job was simply to keep him comfortable and advocate for him to the best of my abilities. But as anyone who's been a caregiver knows, there is very little that is simple in that job description. Too often having to ask, "What hurts?" while being powerless to relieve the pain. Countless appointments. Taking notes. Making phone calls. Asking questions.

Once he came home with that new heart (and the broken hip), my job was to be present and pray through all of it for the grace of God. Provide comfort as best possible. Offer reassurance. Relieve pain. Preserve dignity. Get prescriptions renewed or refilled. Count pills. Then, too often, I found myself arguing with him. (Really? This was us making the best of his new heart?!)

There was an element of guilt before and after the transplant. We suffered from the what-ifs, second-guessed the details we'd missed, regretted the things we'd done and left undone and said and left unsaid. If I'd been paying better attention years earlier, might we have avoided whatever life stresses had triggered the systemic sclerosis? Or the infected ankles that delayed getting him on "the list"? Or the broken hip?

I knew I needed to be rejoicing in the small things. Many people would give anything for the luxury of the time we had before Ben ended up in the hospital. Time to deal. Time to prepare. Time to ask questions. We'd been blessed to have tough conversations regarding what we thought might happen.

And now Ben had a heart! We had our miracle! We had so, so, so much for which to be grateful, and we were so overwhelmed at the challenges still ahead of us.

While he'd been in the hospital, I'd journaled. I'd meditated. And yes, on occasion, I'd medicated. I'd breathed—in and out, in and out—as I closed my eyes at night and before opening them in the morning. Breathing in love, calm, grace, peace, courage, patience (again and again and again), as deeply as possible; breathing out fear, terror, dread, panic, frustration, anger, exhaustion, anxiety, irritation . . . squeezing the last bit of air out of my lungs like water from a sponge so there'd be more room for the positivity of breathing in deeply again.

I was blessed not to be financially challenged in the near term. Whenever that thought crossed my mind, I would resolve to face it if I had to—later.

Once Ben had been discharged from rehab to home and my care, because of the pandemic, it wasn't possible to bring in family and friends to help, and the help being provided by the health-care agencies was so different from what I'd expected and hoped for, I wasn't willing to pursue that option further.

And I found it revealing that through the months and years after his initial diagnosis, Ben took almost every medical development in stride, but it was only once his recovery began that his feelings and frustrations finally came to the fore. Yet his moments of feeling sorry for himself were exceedingly rare, and he never turned bitter or lamented "Why me?" That remains a huge gift and blessing to me and all our family.

Ben was home. Thanks be to God.

I was wiped out physically and emotionally. I needed to find ways to take control. It took me weeks to realize that the most obvious first step in that direction was to roll up my sleeves and learn how to tackle the bedsore myself. Oh, how I did not want to be responsible for that! I'd never had the stomach for blood or wound care, but a new hip was not an option until it was under control. It was only going to get better if I stepped up and learned whatever the professionals were willing to teach me.

And Ben was home. Thanks be to God.

On my own behalf, I continued as best I could. I strived to make time and space for some semblance of normalcy—walks, errands, swimming. I would break the overwhelming tasks into smaller, more manageable bits. I kept lists—all sorts of lists. Things to ask the nurses, the doctors. Stuff to order online. People to call. Emails to send. Thank-yous to say.

Once Ben received the new hip, finally regained his independence, and then passed the six-month-post-transplant milestone, I realized that after so many years of caregiving, it was time to focus on some recovering of my own. After an annual physical, I sat down with a psychologist, Joseph Mora, PhD, who concluded our appointment by noting "You have every reason to be undergoing PTSD—right now, you are the partner in need of repair and healing." He offered basic but lovely advice: "Sleep. Eat right. Exercise when you can. Accept the issues and pains that arise as reality, but too, commit to push on toward what makes life worth living. Establish when and where you need to protect yourself; don't tiptoe; and when it's in your own best interests, let go." He then went on to suggest, "Try to greet the morning with optimistic anticipation, *not* frustration. Ask yourself, 'What gives me pleasure?' Inventory your routines to unearth good and joyous footholds; create them if necessary. Seek avenues to make *each day* better."

In that vein, writing this story of Ben's finding his way back to me has been a powerfully healing exercise.

Ben and I raised our boys in the Episcopal church, but when they became adults, they pushed back on the notion of religion and the concept of a higher power. They reason that human existence is a result of biology and science. But when Ben was in the hospital, I felt all the people who'd ever loved him shining their light from the far reaches of the universe each time I begged them to do so. Whatever doubts the boys may have stirred in my soul in our discussions of faith through the years, all those doubts faded in that all-encompassing love from the universe.

Ben is home. Thanks be to God.

A SMALL FAVOR

If you are already an organ donor, "Way to go, you!"

If you are not, please consider becoming one and letting your loved ones know of your decision.

Thank you. Bless you.

Love bears all things, believes all things,
hopes all things, endures all things.
Love never ends.
—1 Corinthians 13:7–8 ESV

Acknowledgments

It was the love of so many, seen and unseen, every step of the way, that pulled us through. My heartfelt thanks to the host of people who supported us along our journey . . .

My dad—who died in August of 2021 but who in the darkest hours of the five years spanning 2016 through 2020 served as my rock even as his wife, Carol (whose mantra was "Keep having fun!"), faded away. My brother, Rhett, who fought with such grace but lost the good fight in 2018. Several generations of our extended blood family: Austells, Carts, Elorteguis, Jahns, Macauleys, McCartys, Pohlmanns, Straights, Tylers, Ulmers, and Zuills. Our first "family"—the crowd who befriended us and one another in northwestern Massachusetts in the late 1970s: the women of Williams F & Friends (a college dorm in which astoundingly uplifting and lifelong relationships were formed); the men of the Octet and all the Williams College Ephlats; and Dan Chapman, Jon Hammond, MD, and Pete Rowland, DVM, plus the beautiful women those three brought into our lives: Hitomi Chapman, Carrie Hammond, and Jillian Hanson.

The Petrox family, and Mark and Brenda Depew, for their constant care, love, and support through the years and across the miles, plus fellow Depew wedding guest Vivek Thappa, MD. Our extended Poconos family, who have known Ben all his life and welcomed me from the other side of Pike County so many years ago; all Ben's Bermuda relations, and the beloved Bermuda contingent spread across the world who have adopted us as part of their family too, from Tich Montfort to her mother, Fiona Delassus, and Fiona's sisters, Sheila and Moira, and all their clan. Our Ohio friends, for the close bonds they maintained with us through the decades.

The dozens of folks in the Keys who stepped in as surrogate family and called, fed, shared, and cared (unfailingly masked and socially distanced, as the times demanded), including Mona Brewer, RN, and Mary Schlafly (a.k.a. Maria), a precious gem.

On the front lines, the medical miracle workers: Carlos Smith, MD, and the whole team at our community medical center, from the staff at the front desk to the lab technicians to the physical therapists and everyone in between. In Scranton, Thomas Dzwonczyk, MD; Mark Frattali, MD; Daniel Kazmierski, MD; Kristen Maritato, PA-C; Julio Ramos, MD; and Matthew Stopper, MD. Jason Gluck, DO, in Hartford. In Hollywood, Miami, and the Keys, Elizabeth Herrera, MS; Neal Rakov, MD; James Salerno, MD; and Raul Valor, MD. At the Cleveland Clinic Florida, Craig Asher, MD; Nicolas Brozzi, MD; Howard Bush, MD; Hossam Elzawawy, MD; Juan Giraldo, MD; Mazen Hanna, MD; Marcelo Helguera, MD; Luis Hernandez-Mejia, MD; Jaime Hernandez-Montfort, MD; Jorge Manrique, MD; Andres Mascaro, MD; Elsy Navas, MD; Cedric Sheffield, MD; and countless others, including the masked nurses who were already doing so much but bent over backward to facilitate our communications under the toughest of circumstances and whose smiling eyes gave me hope on the roughest days. There were also the therapists, techs, and COVID testers; Mala and the pharmacy crew; and the transplant team, including Deborah Rossignol, RN, and Sophia Wilson, APRN-BC, who continue to support and guide us. And Nurse Connie, for whose work ethic and tutelage we are grateful.

And two men who each stepped in to provide critical assistance late on Saturdays four weeks apart: computer wizard Conal Ryan (when Ben was still at CCF) and the Honorable William W. "Bill" Haury Jr.

(shortly after Ben returned home), plus, for his calm counsel, Atty. Kenneth J. Bush.

Also, for helping me prioritize my own health, trainer Beth Bielat, physical therapist Christine Langley, and for his restorative advice, Joseph Mora, PhD.

As for how to turn all this into a book, I am profoundly grateful for the patience and wisdom of my earliest readers—Barbara Austell, poet Jillian Hanson, Molly Macauley, and Martha Williamson—and to Barbara and Ed Hajim (and Susan Bohan for nudging me in their direction) for the introduction to *New York Times* bestselling author Glenn Plaskin. Glenn, thank you for transforming the proverbial sow's ear. You produced the silk: any porcine remnants or errors are mine alone.

Writing *On My Way Back to You* has been a journey along a steep learning curve, the completion of which would not have been realized without the guidance of the team at Forefront Books and the talents of developmental editor Hope Innelli with her remarkable gift for addressing "the echo effect" (and *so* much more).

As for Ben's and my four amazing sons and our delightfully brilliant grandchildren—you are our greatest blessings and the legacy of our life together. May your hearts be open to miracles.

And lastly, Ben: for all you have taught me about love, endurance, and greeting every situation with openness and faith; for your indomitable spirit, irrepressible resiliance, and Tigger-like energy; for finding your way back to me; and for being my most enthusiastic cheerleader on this project—thank you/bless you. If you would please continue to do so well that you annoy me for decades to come, I will always be grateful—expo expo.